# PESTICIDES
and your
# FOOD

# PESTICIDES
## and your
# FOOD

Andrew Watterson

First published in 1991 by
Green Print
an imprint of The Merlin Press
10 Malden Road, London NW5 3HR

ISBN 1 85425 047 7

1 2 3 4 5 6 7 8 9 10 :: 99 98 97 96 95 94 93 92 91

Phototypeset by Computerset, Harmondsworth

Printed in England by Biddles Ltd., Guildford, Surrey, on recycled paper

# DISCLAIMER

Every effort has been made to ensure that the information in this book is accurate and complete at the time of going to press. However, the author and publishers do not accept liability for any error or omission in the content, and readers are responsible for checking the accuracy and validity of the information before acting upon it.

*The question of chemical residues on the food we eat is a hotly debated issue. The existence of such residues is either played down by industry as unimportant or is flatly denied. Simultaneously, there is a strong tendency to brand as fanatics or cultists all who are so perverse as to demand that their food be free of insect poisons.*

*A laboratory animal, living under controlled and highly artificial conditions, consuming a given amount of a specific chemical, is very different from a human being whose exposures to pesticides are not only multiple but for the most part unknown, unmeasurable and uncontrolled . . . this piling up of chemicals from many different sources creates a total exposure that cannot be measured. It is meaningless to talk about the 'safety' of any specific amount of residue.*

**Rachel Carson** in SILENT SPRING, 1962

*Given today's very extensive use of pesticides, both for agricultural and non-agricultural purposes, it is almost impossible for any member of the population to avoid daily exposure to very low levels of a number of different pesticides in food, water, through skin contact with contaminated surfaces and so on. Consequently there is considerable public concern about possible adverse effects on human health arising from continual long-term exposure, that is chronic exposure. Despite the importance of the problem, it is difficult to provide clear, direct information, either on the impact of such pesticides in toto on human health or indeed the effects of the individual pesticides.*

**House of Commons Select Committee on Agriculture**
REPORT ON THE EFFECTS OF PESTICIDES ON HUMAN HEALTH,
London 1987

# CONTENTS

# ACKNOWLEDGEMENTS

I would like to thank all those who helped in the preparation of this book. They of course are not responsible for how the material has been used or the opinions expressed in the following pages.

I am particularly grateful to Peter Snell and Kirsty Nichol who first started looking closely at the whole area of pesticide residues with the Food Commission and have led the way. I would also like to thank David Seys-Evans for his international food observations and Ann Hayter, Audrey Palmer, Alison Tams, Beverley Williams and Lin White for their invaluable consumer comments on various drafts. My thanks too to Jon Carpenter for giving me the opportunity to write the book and to colleagues at Southampton University for helping to give me a little extra space to get on with it.

Many people have supplied me with information internationally and I would especially like to thank: R.B. Burke, P.R. Bennett and Geraldine Graham of the Health and Welfare Department, Canada and Dr Frank Cedar from Agriculture Canada; Elizabeth Flynn of the Australian Department of Community Services and Health; Torsten Berg of the National Food Agency, Danish Ministry of Health; Juhani Paakkanen of the Finnish Division for Food Affairs; Curtis Coker of the US Food and Drugs Administration; Dr H.P. Bosshart of Switzerland; Dolores Rivas of the Spanish Ministry of Agriculture, Patricia Stolfa of the US Department of Agriculture; Ingegard Bergman of the Swedish National Food Administration; Paulo Miele of the Brazilian Ministry of Health; Max Jaramillo of the Ecuador Ministry of Agriculture; Francis Neri of the Philippines Department of Agriculture; Dr C. Ramcharran, the Guyana Government Analyst; Sylvia Brusewitz of Kemikalienspektiones, Sweden; Dr Topner of the German Ministry of Health; Dr Moshe Hoffman of the Israeli Ministry of Agriculture; Dr Arslan Umit of the Turkish Ministry of Health;

C.W. Fong of the Hong Kong Agriculture Department; D.W. Lunn of the New Zealand Ministry of Agriculture; Dr J. Dabrowski of the Plant Protection Institute in Poland; Avelino Pedro of the Agriculture Ministry, Portugal; Ole Harbitz and Kirstin Faerden of the Norwegian Food Control Authority; Dr Andre Rogirst of the Belgian Ministry of Public Health; and Ms S.H. Leng of the Singapore Food Control Authority.

Finally I would like to thank Jenny for taking far more than her fair share of the domestic burdens during the writing of this book.

# PREFACE

I write this book as someone who believes that fresh vegetables and fresh fruit are important and enjoyable parts of any healthy diet. Readers should not be put off from either continuing or starting such a diet after referring to this book. Fresh vegetables and fruit are much healthier than many processed foods which may contain not only large numbers of the pesticides referred to in this book but also many additional additives and contaminants, fats, salt and sugar.

I live in a house where there are vegetarians, carnivores and fisheaters. I believe that whatever your diet, you have both a need and a right to know how the food you eat has been treated before it reaches you and what chemicals have been used on it in the growing, storage and packaging cycle.

I am firmly convinced that unnecessarily large quantities and types of agro-chemicals are used internationally on livestock, fish, vegetables, cereals and fruit. The produce entries in this book indicate the very wide range of pesticides that can be applied to foods for human consumption and the numbers of residues which have been detected in treated food crops. Consumers should have a right to information both about the effects of those chemicals in the food chain and about the gaps which exist in our knowledge of possible adverse effects.

It is perfectly clear at the moment that we do not fully understand exactly what long-term effects if any low level exposure to a wide range of pesticide residues has upon human populations and sub-populations. In some instances we cannot even detect residues – not because they are absent but because we do not have the technology available to identify them.

The consequences of pesticide use should be viewed not only from the point of view of consumers in Western Europe and North America but also from the point of view of those agricultural workers across the world who have to apply toxic chemicals in difficult conditions, from consumers in developing countries and from the perspective of those concerned with the wider environment and so concerned about the implications of pesticide manufacture, use and disposal in terms of energy consumption, raw materials, contamination from processed products, the effects on water and wildlife and the consequences of waste disposal at the end of the chain. All these elements should be fully discussed and properly audited before any pesticides are cleared for use anywhere in the world.

This book therefore identifies areas of concern and the need for action on a whole range of issues associated with pesticides and food.

# PART 1
# Pesticides and why they are used

## WHAT ARE PESTICIDES?

The term 'pesticide' covers a range of substances used to control pests affecting subsistence or cash crops or human and animal health. Pesticides may be organic products, such as nicotine, or synthetic chemical products, such as paraquat. Pesticides therefore include:-

weedkillers (also known as herbicides)
insecticides or insect pest killers
fungicides (which kill fungi, including mould)
acaricides (which kill spiders)
nematocides (which kill round, thread or eel worms)
rodenticides (which kill mice and rats)
algicides (which kill algae)
miticides (which kill mites)
molluscicides (which kill snails and slugs)
growth regulators (which stimulate or retard plant growth)
defoliants (which remove plant leaves)
desiccants (which speed plant drying)
attractants (which attract insects e.g. pheromones).

Also within this heading come veterinary pesticides and medicinal feed additives. These are only touched on briefly in the following pages, primarily because there is even less publicly available information on them than on pesticide residues.

# WHY ARE PESTICIDES USED?

Pesticides have been used for at least a thousand years. The ancient Greeks, Egyptians and Romans used various forms of pest control including chemicals on a range of insect and fungus pests. Pliny advised applying wine to cereal seed to prevent mildew. Democrates in 470BC used olive extracts to prevent blight on plants while the Chinese used ants as biological controls to protect their trees from insect pests.

Pesticides are used for food production, health protection and weed and fungus control in a wide range of industrial and commercial as well as agricultural settings. Industry frequently argues that there are no real alternatives to large-scale pesticide usage if the food needs and disease control requirements of the world population are to be met. This is a very simplistic argument and smacks of There Is No Alternative (TINA) thinking. Many pesticides have been used on cash crops in the developing world and do not benefit subsistence food production. Sometimes pesticides may be a factor in damaging that subsistence food production through pest resistance and also in creating difficulties in controlling disease vectors like the mosquito. Many people in Western Europe are entirely unconvinced that large agro-chemical inputs are needed to protect food supplies when we have large food surpluses. It is equally a nonsense to suggest that we must have massive agro-chemical inputs in the world to ensure food for the inevitably ever-growing world population. The finite resources of the world indicate that the wise solution lies some-where other than planning for an ever-increasing population.

There are alternatives to large-scale pesticide usage but one would not expect those making chemicals to advocate large-scale integrated pest management programmes and the development of organic farming. But these are alternatives and we shall look at them later.

Although this book is concerned with food use, it should be remembered that pesticides used on non-food pests and crops or disposed of after use may still end up in our water or on our food by a variety of routes. Atrazine for instance appears in water supplies in the UK not because of agricultural use but because some local authorities apply the chemical to control weeds on roads and recreational areas.

# HOW MANY PESTICIDES ARE USED AND HOW MUCH?

Synthetic pesticides have only been used in large quantities in the last forty or fifty years. The US has 1,200 different active ingredients listed for use and some 35,000 pesticide products based on those active ingredients. The World Health Organization (WHO) International Programme on Chemical Safety reports that there are over 1,000 pesticides in over 100,000 commercial formulations used worldwide. In the UK there are several hundred active ingredients available in several thousand trade name products.

Pesticide production and sales are very big global business activities. In 1986 some $13 billion dollars of pesticides were sold in the world and in 1988 the sales of British-Agrochemical Association members totalled just over £1 billion. In 1988 the UK sold 23,504 tonnes of pesticide active ingredient on the home market and 19,600,000 hectares of land were treated with agrochemicals. One estimate is that in the mid-1980s a pound by weight of pesticide was used each year for every person on earth. In the US more than one billion pounds of pesticides by weight were used each year in the 1980s and 79% of that figure was used in agriculture.

# THE EFFECTS ON HUMANS AND THE ENVIRONMENT

Much remains unknown about the effects of pesticides, pesticide mixtures and pesticides mixed with other chemicals or drugs on particular physical conditions and illnesses. There is a lot of controversy surrounding pesticides and their possible effects as carcinogens, mutagens and allergens. There have been many claims and counter-claims about the theory that pesticides at very low levels in food may produce allergic responses. Likewise, we still do not fully understand – and in some instances, have barely started to research – the possibilities of pesticides at very low levels causing changes in the human immune system, damaging human reproductive capacity or adversely affecting our neurological system. Pesticides like paraquat and maneb have been associated with Parkinson's disease but no conclusive evidence is available to prove or disprove a causal link between exposure and disease (Goldsmith 1990).

The consequences of using pesticides have concerned scientists exactly because pesticides are biologically active substances which are deliberately and not accidentally introduced into the environment. This use may then lead to the presence of pesticide residues in food, and the presence of pesticides in water and air.

What is indisputable is that large numbers of pesticides have been detected, albeit often at very low levels, in many foodstuffs sold throughout the world. There have also been a number of epidemics of acute pesticide poisonings in the past due not to low-level residues of pesticide in food but to pesticide spillages or grain treatments. Wales, Egypt, India, Malaya, Turkey, Pakistan, the US and several other countries have all experienced such pesticide food poisoning epidemics. In Wales, flour contaminated by endrin caused 159 poisoning cases; in Qatar such flour caused 691 poisonings and 24 deaths. Parathion in wheat poisoned 360 and killed 120 and the same chemical in flour poisoned 600 and killed 88 in Colombia. In Turkey the consumption of seed grain treated with HCB poisoned over 3,000 and between 3-11% of those died.

By 1969, 17 pesticide food epidemics had been recorded (E. M. Mrak, USFDHEW 1969). The effects of acute poisoning are relatively easy to diagnose and record: the effects of low-level exposure are not.

The US has one of the better records on monitoring pesticides and yet even there the information available is far from complete. Some 496 pesticides can potentially leave residues on or in food yet of these only 316 in the USA had tolerances (or control standards or MRLs) set. In 1987, of the 316 pesticides with tolerances set, only 41% could be detected by multiple residue testing at the time. There is some evidence to suggest that even for pesticides with tolerances, the regulatory agencies still lack the data needed to determine safe residue levels.

It will take many years in most countries to assess those pesticides cleared in the past when testing standards were less complete and rigorous than they are now. An indication of the serious nature of the gaps came in 1984 when the US General Accounting Office (GAO) found that of 92 pesticides in one of its studies, 62% had data gaps on tumours and 73% had data gaps on birth defects. (Source: Summary information from US GAO on pesticides prepared by Dr Marion Moses, July 1987).

Peter Snell, a UK food technologist, looked at 426 pesticides cleared in the UK in the 1980s and found 68 were possible carcinogens, 61 were possible mutagens, 35 had been linked with reproductive effects and a further 93 were known irritants. This indicates a real cause for concern. Some scientists think that pesticides at low levels are a causal factor in several diseases and may be linked to food chemical sensitivity: others do not. (Bust 1986: 132-155).

One important consideration for consumers in these global green times must now be the human and environmental costs of certain pesticide usage on crops in Africa, Asia and South America and exported for food to Western Europe and North America. The more conservative estimates suggest that worldwide there are hundreds of thousands of cases of pesticide poisoning and tens of thousands of deaths from pesticide exposure. One estimate from the WHO/UN Environment Programme indicates that there could be up to one million cases of unintentional poisonings from pesticides each year. In countries like Sri Lanka, the Philippines and other Central American and South East Asian states, occupational and environmental health problems created by pesticide usage are now major causes of illness and death (Watterson 1988: 24-25 and Loevinsohn 1987).

The main pesticide chemical groups have known acute effects and sometimes either unknown or potentially serious chronic effects.

**Organophosphorous** insecticides are neurotoxic and have affected the human nervous system and may cause protracted peripheral neuropathy. Others have been linked to mutagenicity and animal carcinogenicity.

**Organochlorines** have caused concern because of their long-term persistence in the environment, storage in body fat and carcinogenicity in test animals. They can also interfere with the metabolism of chemicals and can affect the nervous system at high doses.

**Chlorophenoxy herbicides** have been linked with potential carcinogenicity, neurological effects and teratogenicity. (Fan and Jackson 1989).

In terms of human toxicity, organic or natural does not of course necessarily mean safe, as readers will realize from the reference to nicotine as an organic insecticide. Nor does synthetic necessarily mean harmful.

In the early 1960s, William Hupert, a professor of medicine and a specialist in oncology, expressed concern to Rachel Carson about the potential long-term problems of pesticides and human cancer. Thirty years on, a number of medical observers echo those concerns, especially Professor Samuel Epstein, a toxicologist at the University of Illinois. There is much debate about the causes of cancer and the role played by environmental factors. One school of thought takes the view that synthetic pollutants which include chemicals in drinking water and pesticide residues in food pose minimal carcinogenic risks to humans relative to the background of natural carcinogens (Ames and others, *Science,* 17 April 1987). Others like Epstein believe that this is not the case. Epstein argues persuasively that natural carcinogens may be influenced by harvesting and storage technology and nitrite additives; that natural anticarcinogens and antimutagens in our diet have been ignored in the past; that the increase of synthetic carcinogens in our environment, unlike the natural carcinogens which have always played a part in human cancer, must be a focus for current concerns. Epstein observes that:

> Growing evidence demonstrates that pervasive contamination of air, water, soil and food with a wide range of industrial carcinogens, generally without public knowledge and consent, is important in causation of modern preventable cancer. Even if hazards posed by any industrial carcinogen are small, their cumulative, possibly synergistic [combined effect being greater than single chemical effect] effects are likely to be substantial. Eating food contaminated with residues at maximum legal tolerances of only 28 of 53 known carcinogenic pesticides, excluding numerous other carcinogenic pesticides and incremental exposure in drinking water, is estimated to be potentially responsible for 1.5 million excess lifetime US cancers. (*Science,* 20 May 1988: 1044).

The balance of probabilities approach has some value in this debate. If Ames is correct, there is little to worry about in the levels of pesticide residues recorded in food; but if he is not, and Epstein is correct, the consequences for many people could be disastrous. Many believe that if we assume the worst and regulate chemicals with great circumspection, we protect ourselves much better.

Some scientists have noted that there may be extensive mixing of pesticide residues due to consumption of many foods which could have been treated with a wide range of different pesticides. It has been assumed that such mixed residues would not be particularly toxic but in the mid-1980s work had not been done to establish the facts and test that assumption. In 1981 the JMPR noted that pesticides and other chemical compounds to which people were exposed could interact and very little data on these reactions was available. The Joint Meeting on Pesticide Residues (JMPR) is the most powerful international body which sets maximum residue limits of pesticides in food commodities. It consists of the Food and Agriculture Organisation (FAO) Panel of Experts on Pesticide Residues in Food and the World Health Organization (WHO) Expert Group on Pesticides Residues. With the low level of pesticide residue intake, JMPR felt that there was no particular concern over such interactions. They did encourage the development of knowledge of combined toxic effects in pesticide residues 'in view of the possible toxicological interactions that can arise from pesticide mixtures' (JMPR 1981 cited in Gibson and Walker by Parke and others). Again there is no denial from scientists that there were gaps in our knowledge, but the debate relates to the significance of those gaps.

Those who study patterns of disease, epidemiologists, have great difficulty in taking into account all the factors which might explain the trends in cancer mortality and morbidity. Many such studies produce negative results but this does not mean that they have proved chemicals do not cause cancer; rather, that the information available and methods used simply do not allow any meaningful conclusions to be drawn. Recently a number of epidemiologists have published research which links occupational exposure to pesticides with cancer mortality in a number of countries but again it is difficult to draw meaningful conclusions from the work. No one knows exactly or even roughly what effect many pesticides have on human health at very low levels. One can only speculate.

A recent report in *The Lancet* described cancer mortality trends in West Germany, Italy, Japan, the US and England and Wales. The report found that brain cancer, central nervous system cancers, breast cancer, multiple myeloma, kidney cancer, non-Hodgkins lymphoma and melanoma were all increasing in people of 55 and older. Such trends remain unexplained but one might fairly speculate that a range of environmental factors could be involved. The authors themselves touch on smoking, dirty workplaces, lower consumption of fresh fruit and vegetables, medical radiation and poor control of newly introduced household pesticides and chemicals in the 1940s and 1950s as possible factors in increased cancer risks for the group in question (Lee, Davis, Hoel, Fox and Lopez, in *The Lancet*, 25 August 1990: 480).

Other doctors, such as Richard Mackarness (*Chemical Victims*, Pan Books, 1980), have raised the question of chemicals, including pesticides, causing allergies at very low levels in those exposed either at work, in the general environment or through food. Dr J. R. Mansfield has pointed out that food allergy and the approach of clinical ecologists to it is a very recent development and the part played by pesticide residues, if any, in most allergies is still very unclear (Mansfield 1983 in Conning and Lansdown).

The US Environmental Protection Agency's National Human Monitoring programme began to sample human fatty tissue in 1970 and has, in conjunction with other agencies, been looking at pesticides in the blood and urine of the general population. In 1983 the programme found 99% of all subjects tested had detectable DDT in blood samples; approximately 80% had detectable levels of pentachlorophenol in their urine and 2%-4% had carbamate pesticide metabolites. The figures for various organophosphorous residues in urine ranged from 6%-12%. Organochlorine residues have also been widely detected in human milk across the world (Coye 1986).

In the light of our ignorance about the exact effects of pesticides on humans it would seem both wise and reasonable to allow consumers a right to basic information about possible residues in food or, as many pesticide residues are not monitored in many foods and as some pesticides still cannot be tested for, the right to know what pesticides have been applied to the food crops that they may wish to eat.

Studies of consumer attitudes to pesticides outside the UK suggest that people are less worried about pesticides causing cancer than about pesticides causing allergies or learning disorders which might affect children (*Pesticide and Toxic Chemicals News,* 6 June 1990).

The effect of pesticide residues on wildlife has received a great deal of attention since the work of Rachel Carson and others. The problems of persistent organochlorine exposure for birds and marine life has been documented in detail and highlighted the inability of scientists to forecast the chronic effects of pesticides at extremely low levels in the environment. These residues have built up through the food chain with disastrous consequences for birds of prey. Problems have emerged for fish, shellfish and coral exposed to extremely low doses of pesticides in their environment either due to run-off or spray drift or spillage. It is also clear that we do not fully understand the implications of pesticide application and later soil erosion and water contamination. In the UK the complex effects spraying has on birds in terms of habitat loss or loss of either insect food, cover or plant foods is now only just being realized. One wonders again about the extent to which we are gambling with our world on the basis of ignorance.

# HOW PESTICIDES ARE CONTROLLED

## Toxicology

The methods used to calculate exactly what are safe levels of chemicals, be they pesticides or food additives, in our food are yet again subjects of controversy. Some scientists argue that past screening of pesticides, concentrating on identifying animal carcinogens, has been expensive, time-consuming and of little value to the process of predicting the risks to humans from such chemicals. Others argue that our knowledge of human and animal toxicology is incomplete and more and fuller tests should be carried out before pesticides are cleared. Between these points lie a range of views.

The basic approach is to test new chemicals in a variety of ways, principally on laboratory animals. This immediately raises an issue which we should not ignore: namely the ethics of animal testing. It may be argued that pesticides need to be developed to control insects spreading diseases, to safeguard subsistence crop production or to take account of new climatic or ecological changes on crops. Significant parts of the agro-chemical market are devoted to cash crop production and not to subsistence farming. I do not believe that the development of new pesticides tested on animals is justified if alternative tests are available and if there is no major health or subsistence food need for the new pesticides. In these circumstances the ethics of animal testing should perhaps loom larger than it does in the debates.

At the moment the risk assessment of pesticides is still based on toxicology. Groups of animals are exposed to a pesticide usually in their diet, but sometimes through skin absorption or a combination of routes of entry.

The animals are exposed to the chemical over a lifetime and the maximum level to which they can be exposed without adverse effects is called the 'no observable effect level' (NOEL) or sometimes the 'no observable adverse effect level' (NOAEL).

You may of course get observable effects which are not regarded as adverse: hence the NOEL and the NOAEL are not necessarily one and the same thing. Exactly what constitutes an adverse effect as opposed to a normal biological response is determined by groups of scientists. In the US such scientists have on occasions disagreed about the interpretation of laboratory evidence: some have said that given pesticides have caused cancers in animals and others have not.

## Regulatory practices

Regulatory practices at the moment are based on a number of key concepts and use the following key terms which are defined below.

**The Maximum Residue Level (MRL)** is defined as the maximum concentration of a pesticide residue – usually measured in mg/kg but in some countries referred to in ppm – which is legally permitted in or on food commodities and animal feed. These MRLs are based on the adoption of good agricultural practice (see below). In addition it is intended that foods derived from commodities which comply with the MRLs will be toxicologically acceptable.

**The Acceptable Daily Intake (ADI)** is the amount of a pesticide which can be consumed every day for an individual's entire lifetime in the practical certainty, on the basis of all the known facts, that no harm will result. The ADI is expressed as mg of the chemical per kg of body weight of the consumer. The ADI is based on the toxicological 'no effect' level in the most sensitive animal species, or for people if appropriate data are available. It includes a safety factor to account for variations in responses between species and variations in human responses. Studies from which NOELs and hence ADIs are derived are conducted with the technical pesticide so that any toxic effects of impurities in the pesticide will be included in the assessment. Account is also taken of any degradation or break-down products (metabolites) which may affect the toxicity of the residue reaching the consumer.

The ADI is usually 100 times lower than the NOEL and is calculated on the basis that animal susceptibility may be 10 times greater than that observed in the animals in the test, and that human susceptibility may vary and be up to 10 times greater than that allowed for under normal circumstances. (Hence $10 \times 10 = 100$ and the ADI figure is established). In some instances, however, the ADI set is much lower than this. ADIs should include consideration of short-term and long-term tests, tests for carcinogenicity, mutagenicity, reproductive hazards, teratogenicity as well as general pharmacological and biochemical effects and modes of action.

**Good Agricultural Practice (GAP)** with regard to the use of chemicals relates to the nationally authorised safe uses of pesticides under the conditions necessary for effective and reliable pest control. It covers a range of pesticide applications up to the highest authorised use but applied in a manner which leaves a residue which is the smallest practicable. Authorized safe uses relate to national controls and registered recommended uses which take account of occupational, environmental and public safety considerations. (The above definitions are based on, but not identical in all respects to, those cited in the British MAFF WPPR report (HMSO 1990: iv)).

In the UK, *Guidance Notes on Crop Residue Data Collection and Presentation* issued under the 1986 Control of Pesticides Regulations by the Ministry of Agriculture, Fisheries and Food (MAFF) identify the need for the identification of residues produced in a crop including metabolites, degradation and conversion products; an analytical method to identify the residues; details on residue behaviour in the crop; the problem of residues bound into crops (see the entry for Bread in Part 2); sampling methods; effects of peeling, trimming and cooking; sampling processed products; animal feed studies; and the extrapolation of the residue data for other crop varieties grown under different climatic conditions and/or cultivation methods. It is difficult to obtain such data and rarely in the UK or US do full data exist on the residue chemistry of most pesticides cleared prior to 1985.

Different models have guided the regulatory approaches of different countries both in dealing with the approval of pesticides generally and in dealing with the specific problems presented by pesticide residues. Some models are based on the *balance of probabilities* approach and others are based on the *beyond reasonable doubt* approach (Watterson 1982). The 'balance of probabilities' approach comes from the civil law concept and requires a lower level of proof – on the balance of probabilities – that a pesticide might present harm to humans or the environment. The approach is the most cautious, most conservative and builds in the biggest safety margins to chemical hazards. The policy explains some of the differences between the way Scandinavian countries regulate pesticides and the way the UK and, to a lesser extent, the US have controlled them (Watterson 1990a). The 'beyond reasonable doubt' approach requires a higher level of proof before action is taken to control or remove a chemical hazard.

The problem with the latter approach for a number of environmentalists and scientists is that sometimes by the time the proof is satisfactory and is beyond reasonable doubt a potentially toxic chemical could have been used among workers and affected the environment and the public for many years; the consequences could be irreversible. With hindsight it is possible to identify chemicals which do not meet current health and safety standards and for which there was balance of probability evidence in the past: asbestos, several bladder carcinogens and a number of pesticides would appear to fall into this category.

In the US the control of pesticide residues is dealt with differently as Congress interpreted the Delaney provision of the Food Insecticide, Fungicide and Rodenticide Act. The US approach, simply put, meant that where the cost of a false negative was high (allowing through a carcinogen into the food supply when the benefits of such a carcinogen were small against even a few extra cancers in the population) when compared with the cost of a false positive (banning a substance which was not a carcinogen), it was wise to have a system which tripped easily and allowed fewer false negatives than positives (Page and Robbins

1981). The Delaney clause is intended to apply a zero-risk standard on potential carcinogens in food.

This indicates the value of a broad cost-benefit approach to pesticide regulation which sadly has still not been adopted worldwide. There has been a reluctance on the part of the pesticide manufacturers and some governments to disclose the data on pesticide testing and registration which fully evaluate the costs of producing, using and disposing of pesticides as against the benefits of use. A few US medical practitioners have looked at it, but the full auditing of pesticides has not been done, at least publicly, in the UK. One can imagine that the benefits from some pesticides would be minimal at a time of over-production and food surplus in Western Europe.

The difficulty with the US approach to carcinogens in food and pesticide residues is that newer pesticides may pose much less of a risk than older pesticides which were not so carefully screened. Yet the newer chemicals may not gain clearance because they show evidence of oncogenicity in the new tests which the older pesticides did not go through. Hence the newer pesticides trip the regulatory safeguard system of no carcinogens in food. Perhaps there is an argument here for not clearing any suspect carcinogens and devoting resources less to new pesticide development and more to integrated and biological pest control methods?

The National Research Council (NRC) was approached by the Environmental Protection Agency (EPA) in 1985 to look at the very complex methods used for regulating pesticide residues in food in that country. The outcome was *Regulating Pesticides in Food: the Delaney Paradox* (National Academy Press, Washington DC, 1987). This is undoubtedly the most detailed examination of the issue of pesticides in food. The NRC attempted to quantify the oncogenic risk from pesticide residues in particular foods in the US – the so-called Q star factor, calculated by assuming residues were all at the tolerance level or the highest level allowed; that the calculations would look at body weight, surface area, extrapolation of risks from rodents to humans, exposure to a range of foodstuffs and so on. (Oncogens are those substances which can cause malignant or benign tumours in animals.) The report stresses, unlike other approaches, the wide margin of uncertainty in these calculations and the fact that only oncogenic effects of pesticide residues were being examined. The EPA regulates oncogenic pesticides using qualitative evidence like tumour types in animals, mutagenicity bioassays and general toxicological evidence as well as now taking note of the quantitative methods outlined here.

The NRC identified 53 oncogenic pesticides used on US crops, on the basis of EPA research. They then looked at the dietary risks from 28 of those pesticides. They found that fungicides accounted for about 60% of the dietary oncogenic risk from the 28 pesticides; herbicides and then insecticides were next in importance. The committee also found that about 55% of the total estimated dietary oncogenic risk stemmed from residues on crops that had raw and processed food forms. Details of the potential oncogens identified in the NRC report are incorporated into the toxicity section of this book. The EBDCs were identified as a major group of fungicides presenting a significant oncogenic risk. The risk figures relate to disease incidence estimates and not to estimates of deaths. They are of course calculations and not recorded cases.

Recently efforts have been made by those scientists in the UK who advise the government on pesticide approvals to publicise the basis of their decision-making (Advisory Committee on Pesticides (ACP), *Annual Report 1988:* HMSO 1990: 29-34). Their approach is geared far more to understanding the toxicology of pesticides and the models of pesticide action in animals through the pharmacokinetics and pharmacodynamics, rather than on quantitative risk assessment models. They feel that the toxicology and not the more theoretical areas of statistics provide the best risk assessments of pesticides. In some respects this policy mirrors that of the WHO IPC Environmental Criteria Document on *The Principles for the Toxicological Assessment of Pesticide Residues in Food* (WHO Geneva, 1990). The ACP note the need to identify the nature and quantity of residues in food, the need to take note of data from epidemiological studies in humans and the importance, in the absence of details on the toxic effects of the pesticide in people, of using appropriate animal studies and extrapolating the results obtained to people. This approach also makes a major distinction between the hazards presented by genotoxic carcinogens and those presented by epigenetic ones. (Genotoxic carcinogens interfere with the genetic information in the cell; epigenetic carcinogens do not affect cell genetic information). The former are viewed as much more hazardous than the latter. Some scientists, perhaps the majority, feel that thresholds can be set for epigenetic carcinogens; others are less sanguine and believe there may even be problems identifying exactly what is an epigenetic carcinogen.

In Britain, the Ministry of Agriculture, Fisheries and Food (MAFF) uses data from sources like the National Food Survey and information on food consumed outside the home to estimate pesticide intake and work out how much the extreme consumer of certain foods would eat.

Frederica Perera has suggested that too much emphasis has been placed on quantitative risk assessments and cost-benefit analyses of toxic chemicals and pesticides. This then disguises the value judgements and uncertainties which underlie regulatory decisions. She favours risk assessments which acknowledge the data gaps in pesticide toxicology and which recognize to a greater extent than has hitherto been the case the varied responses of humans to chemical exposure (Perera 1987). Such an approach again has much to commend it in setting cautious standards which fail to safety more quickly than existing regulation in many countries.

The World Health Organization criteria document on pesticide residue assessment and testing makes specific reference to the lack of standard tests on immunotoxicity and neurotoxicity throughout the 1980s. The criteria relating to existing tests have not been sufficiently developed to be of value in routine safety assessments. The value judgements and data gaps implicit in such evaluation of pesticide residues hinted at by Perera are helpfully identified by the WHO in its 1990 residue document.

# PESTICIDE RESIDUES AND HOW THEY ARE MONITORED

Small residues of a pesticide treatment or the decomposition products (or metabolites) of a pesticide may remain after the treatment of a plant or animal; or they may be absorbed into the plant or animal accidentally through water, air or soil pesticide contamination from spray drift or previous applications. As the *World Directory of Pesticide Control Organisations* observed, 'since food is not labelled as treated with pesticides and these residues are usually only detected by the most sophisticated analytical techniques, the consumer has little option but to accept this involuntary risk' (RSC 1989: 4). The Directory goes on to point out that good agricultural practice should mean that such residues are very small and those government controls that exist should ensure that there is no health risk to consumers. However, the measurement, control and effect of pesticide residues are areas of much controversy.

In the UK, MAFF stresses that not all pesticides leave residues or leave residues at anything other than extremely low and therefore insignificant levels in terms of human health (Pesticides and Food: a balanced view, MAFF, 1990). We have, however, already raised questions about our ability to identify all the pesticides to which we may be exposed and our capacity to assess the effects of that exposure.

The analytical chemists who carry out residue analysis – and these may be commercial, government or, in the case of the UK, public analysts – need to do three things in their work. They separate out the chemicals in a sample, identify them, and then measure the quantities of chemicals they have identified. All three tasks are demanding, especially steps two and three.

Dr Marion Moses indicated that multiple residue testing will not pick up a significant number of pesticides and this raises the question of the extent to which we know the full degree of our exposure to pesticide residues. Helmu Frehse of Bayer noted in 1987 that there were many pesticides and metabolites which could not be determined at all by multi-residue tests (in Greenhalgh 1987). Dr Molly Coye found that in 1986 the US Food and Drugs Administration's most commonly used multi-residue test could identify and quantify only 93 of the 300 pesticides registered at the time for use on food; other residue testing could identify an additional 57 pesticides. This meant that 150 pesticides would not regularly be identified and multi-residue tests in that period would only identify around 33% of the pesticide residues which could occur in food. The methods for identifying pesticide residues in human tissue are even more restricted; in the mid-1980s the US, again among the leaders in the field, could identify only approximately 38 pesticides in body tissues (*Journal of Public Health Policy* 1986, 7: 344).

One example from a Canadian residue analyst will perhaps illustrate the problem and indicate how selective and narrow our knowledge of pesticide residues could be either by design or by accident. Multi-residue tests cannot detect and measure all pesticides, or even all pesticides in a single class of compounds. The analyst must therefore have some knowledge or 'instinct' for the pesticides which may be present in a particular food or water supply. The Canadian laboratory was asked to analyse a US well for alachlor contamination. They decided to use a multi-residue test which allowed them to identify many triazines and chloroacetamide herbicides as well as alachlor. Their results showed triazine and alachlor contamination of the well. If they had not done this test or had been asked to test just for alachlor, the contamination picture of the well would have been very incomplete (Brian Ripley in Greenhalgh 1987).

The testing of pesticide residues is undoubtedly expensive, time-consuming and requires specialist equipment involving gas liquid and high performance liquid chromatography and mass spectrophotometers for water as well as food samples. All the foods consumed in a country cannot be tested. All processed food cannot be monitored, even though we know that some pesticides and their degradation products will survive cooking and processing; some may become more concentrated while others will become much less concentrated.

Those responsible for residue testing are therefore selective in what they test and how they test. In the best approach, foods will be selected for random testing which are both raw and processed, which may have been treated with the more toxic chemicals, and are imports from countries with weaker regulations. In addition, foods should be tested from typical 'household' food baskets and from diets of the not-so-typical but perhaps more vulnerable consumers in any society. This would mean looking particularly at the diets of the very young, the very old, the sick, pregnant women, ethnic minorities, vegetarians and others with special or atypical diets. Such an approach also raises the question about how representative a typical food basket is, what criteria have been used to select it, and how widely and thoroughly the basket has been checked for a very wide range of pesticides indeed. EPA and Natural Resources Defense Council (NRDC) risk estimates on Alar, the growth regulator daminozide, considered not only lifetime exposure to this chemical but also the possible greater vulnerability of the very young to chemicals through their physiological development, lower weight and chemical detoxification processes.

The 1990 Annual Report of the Working Party on Pesticide Residues (WPPR), which tests for residues in some 3,000 UK food samples per year, reported analyses of 667 samples of fruit and vegetables for up to 37 different pesticide residues. This resulted in an analysis of 12,107 individual pesticide/crop combinations. Residues were found in 26% of the samples. Five per cent of the samples tested contained residues over the MRL in fruit, vegetables and rice as well as wood pigeon and Chinese rabbit meat. Residues were found in 22% of the bread sampled in 1989; organochlorines were found in 12% of the retail milk sampled for the same year.

There is some value in looking at how different countries tackle residue testing. The UK does not have either the worst or the best testing policy and practice. For instance, in much smaller Norway approximately 2,000 samples of food were tested in 1989 for 28 different pesticides and 0.6% contained residues over Norwegian MRLs. However, the Norwegians aim to be testing 4,000 samples by 1993/4 for approximately 130 different compounds. California routinely monitors for 67 pesticide residues and in 1986 found residues in 14% of the 4,601 commodities it tested. Belgium between 1985 and 1990 found, through multi-residue testing that 8% to 12% of the food crops it analysed exceeded permitted standards and between 9% and 18% exceeded EBDC or inorganic bromide levels. Sweden tested 4,374 fresh fruit and vegetable samples in 1989 for 209 pesticides, detected 91 different pesticides and found that 3.2% exceeded its control standards. In the US in 1988 the FDA sampled 18,000 domestic and imported foodstuffs for 256 pesticides and detected 118 pesticides in the samples. Between 1979 and 1985 the FDA monitored 67,500 domestic samples and found that 2.9% contained illegal pesticide residues; in the same period the FDA tested 33,690 imported samples and found that 6.1% contained illegal pesticide residues.

If you cannot or do not look for a large number of the pesticide residues, it is no surprise that you do not find them or are not in a position to state whether they are present or not. There is a considerable difference in a monitoring policy which looks for 28 pesticide residues rather than 256 and tests 667 food samples rather than 4,300.

The UK Select Committee on Agriculture raised doubts about the adequacy of residue monitoring in the 1980s and also noted that better methods of residue analysis were needed. Only in the last few years has the government in the UK adopted MRLs and by 1990 there were fewer than a hundred in force. Other standards based on CAC and EC MRLs are used as guidance but the UK is certainly not in the lead in setting standards in Europe, never mind the world, to control pesticide residues. Britain has called for a more open regulatory system. Peter Snell writing in *The Ecologist* (19; 3. 1989) noted that the MAFF Residues Report for 1985 to 1988 found that 43% of fruit and vegetables tested in that period contained detectable residues and 29% had residues over the MRLs. A survey by public analysts found that 1.3% of the products they tested contained residue levels above the MRLs. Some would interpret these and the figures quoted above from the WPPR as not entirely satisfactory.

A major worry in the UK and other countries must relate to the issues of minimum harvest intervals (the time between pesticide application and harvest) and application rates which link into good agricultural practice. If large numbers of fruit and vegetables are never tested for residues, or the tests cannot detect pesticides which may have been applied, it becomes even more important that good agricultural practice is enforced. There are insufficient Health and Safety Executive (HSE) inspectors in Britain to visit farms and enforce the regulations on pesticides.

The likelihood of a health and safety farm visit coinciding with a farmer breaching application rates on pesticide use would appear to be remote. Even more remote would be the possibility that the HSE inspector would be in a position to pick up the infringement unless she or he was standing over the farmer during application of the pesticide. How, exactly, anyone is meant to enforce effectively the minimum harvest interval is even more unclear. There has been just one report of two actions on crop contamination linked to harvest intervals by the HSE up to 1990 and this was due to information from informants and not from enforcement officers. One can only speculate how many other breaches of the laws and good agricultural practice there may be which lead to crops being sold with residues above the MRL.

# ALTERNATIVES TO HIGH PESTICIDE USE

Information and labelling is the key for consumer action on pesticides. This will permit the 'informed consumer' to choose which foods are purchased containing which pesticides if any. The right to know (or the right to be told that no one knows the effects of, or can monitor, or has monitored, the pesticides used on a food crop) would seem to most people to be a basic human right.

Those who argue that concern about environmental health issues is all too often the result of scaremongering pressure groups or unscientific opinions have a great responsibility to disclose full information about topics such as pesticide residues. Some agro-chemical industry spokespersons and scientists are already arguing that the risk from pesticide residues in food is trivial and some scientists argue that valuable resources should not be wasted on monitoring and researching carcinogenic risks from pesticides further.

If this is really the case, the consumer would be forgiven for assuming that all the research has been done to assess fully the effects of pesticide residues in food and that such research has been published, scrutinized and found convincing. Unfortunately there is no evidence to support that case. The areas of ignorance sketched out above *do* exist. Yet again we have the case of industry, sometimes government and some scientists arguing that the absence of evidence of adverse human health effects from pesticide residues is evidence of the absence of such risks. This is simply not so.

Scientists disagree about pesticide health and safety but such disagreements tend to remain unpublicized. Where the disputes are publicized, efforts have on occasions been made to label scientists dissenting from the industry or government view as 'cranks and troublemakers' (Van den Bosch 1978). Sadly the history of environmental and occupational health shows that such 'cranks and troublemakers' can get it right and, on occasions, the industry and scientific establishment can get it woefully wrong. Asbestos and lead spring readily to mind as examples, closely followed by radiation, greenhouse gases and food poisoning.

The other remarkable thing about some of those scientists who believe the hazards posed by pesticide residues to be exaggerated is that they do so on grounds which will greatly, and I think rightly, increase public doubt and scepticism. For instance, some scientists have assured us for many years that they fully understood how toxins in food worked, how many toxins there were in food and what effect they would have on humans. They assured us that they could test for carcinogens and mutagens.

Surprisingly the public is now being told that many foods contain natural carcinogens that were there all the time and that these carcinogens present a much greater hazard than any synthetic carcinogens developed for use as pesticides by industry. Something doesn't quite fit here. Either industry could test crops and identify carcinogens in the past or it could not. The claims about the recent discovery of natural carcinogens in crops appear to destroy a good deal of the credibility of 'science' being able to identify and assess the past existence of carcinogens, natural or otherwise in our food! Perhaps a simpler explanation would be that the food and agriculture industries knew about natural carcinogens in food but did not wish to inform the public about the matter for fear of food scares and chemophobia.

It is difficult to understand how keeping people in ignorance will establish or maintain public confidence in industry or governments on any issue. Indeed, many believe that such a policy has exactly the opposite effect and its past use is rebounding badly on those who used it.

Now we are being told by some scientists that the toxicological methods used in the past to assess the long-term hazards of chemicals to humans has created 'phantom hazards' which require expensive clean-up solutions, that the 'resultant stringent regulation' led to 'public anxiety and chemophobia' and that 'real hazards' are not receiving adequate attention. No information is given about what the 'real hazards' are or how the risks from them have been quantified (Philip Abelson in *Science,* 21 September 1990).

How exactly can such an approach be interpreted? If the scientists got pesticide regulation woefully wrong in the past, on what basis should the public now have greater confidence in them? If the models for risk assessment in the past were deficient, on what basis should we accept their new risk assessment models? We are told that 27 rodent carcinogens naturally present in food have been found out of 52 tested chemicals naturally occurring in food. These 27 carcinogens have been found in 57 different foods including apples, bananas, carrots, celery, coffee, lettuce, orange juice, peas, potatoes and tomatoes. We are also told that they are present in quantities thousands of times greater than synthetic pesticides.

The wisest policy must surely be to cease to take uninformed or ill-informed decisions about the possible health ill-effects of the synthetic chemicals that we use. We should remove or reduce our exposure to carcinogens, allergens, immunotoxic and neurotoxic agents as much as we can. This means surely that we should not be adding more synthetic carcinogens to our food than is absolutely necessary, despite (or because of!) the existence of natural carcinogens in the food already.

The concept of the prudent pessimist has been around for several years and has recently been taken up again by David Pearce in *A Blueprint for a Green Economy*. Prudent pessimists are those who do not accept the assurances of the technological optimists. These optimists are committed to large-scale growth and development in the belief that their models and forecasts and calculations of the consequences are certain to be true. If the technological optimists have it right, there is nothing to worry about. If they have got it wrong, disaster could follow. The prudent pessimists do not believe that society must stagnate and that science and technology should be set aside for some mystical and romantic rural utopia. Rather they believe that we should use science and technology but build in bigger safeguards for our environment and ourselves; hence the costs of a miscalculation will not be disaster.

The approach of this book is very much that of the prudent pessimist.

## Integrated Pest Management (IPM)

Assumptions are often made that there is no alternative to pesticide use and so we must put up with the occupational and environmental health risks attached to agro-chemicals. This is simply not the case. Nor is it correct to assume that pesticides are the 'traditional' method of controlling pests on farms, in parks and gardens. Historically pesticides are a very new development indeed. Before the 1940s, pesticides were used relatively little, so there have always been alternatives to synthetic pesticides. The debate concerns the effectiveness of those alternatives in the light of current world food demands and requirements for vector-borne disease control. (Vectors are animals, usually insects, that transmit diseases to other creatures. Mosquitoes, for example, are vectors of malaria.)

The organic approach which is based on 'natural methods' of pest control does not require the use of any 'artificial' pesticides. Organic farming has been practised for millennia, developed further by farmers recently in several countries, and has been highly successful. Public opinion may lead to even greater pressure for this type of farming.

One study has recently indicated that Britain's cereal growers could cut their energy input, in the form of their use of pesticides and fertilisers, by up to 70%, create several thousand new agricultural jobs by organic rather than chemical farming methods and materials, yet still produce almost the same cereal yields as at present (Pimentel et al, 1983, 359-372).

How carefully and thoroughly the organic and Integrated Pest Management (IPM) options are investigated and, where effective, promoted depends very much on government policies. In the UK, state and academic funding for such work is extremely limited and, until very recently, was almost non-existent. In Germany and Sweden the picture is very different with much work now going on into the possible alternatives to chemical agricultural methods.

The only real criticisms that are levelled against organic farming are that it is not as efficient or profitable as chemical farming. Even this is being questioned in the traditional British agricultural press (*Farmers Weekly*, 21 October 1983). Elsewhere in the world insect pest problems are likely to be greater and human populations may be near starvation. In such circumstances the organic philosophy may be difficult to apply so quickly, completely and successfully. This means and has meant that outside Western Europe IPM has been more widely used than pure organic farming.

## What is Integrated Pest Management?

It is a combination of pest control methods which does not rely solely or, in some instances, at all on the use of agro-chemicals. The methods are based on an understanding of the pest problem in the full environmental context. The approach is therefore an 'ecological' one.

The following elements exist in IPM. The list is not exhaustive, nor would all the elements need to be applied or applied at the same time.

(1) *Biological control* Well over 200 examples exist of the introduction of successful natural predator control of insects. The most common example of biological control in Britain is probably that of aphids by ladybirds. In the western US in the 1950s, beetles were used to control weeds. In Barbados in the 1960s parasites were used to control the citrus fly. Biological control can also include conservation and augmentation of the pest's natural enemies through the provision of food and habitat for the beneficial predator. Such natural biological control can produce high economic returns. (The introduction of non-indigenous pest predators can create unforeseen hazards, however, and may not provide the most effective solution to pest control. Such predators can disrupt local ecological stability with unfortunate and considerable food and economic consequences).

(2) *Cultural control* This entails 'good farming practices' based on traditional methods: for example, the removal of crop residues by ploughing, flooding, long leys and hoeing; inter-planting crops with beneficial covers; pest deterrents and trap crops; the planting of a variety of crops; crop rotation; improved drainage (and filling in low spots to remove mosquito breeding grounds).

(3) *Physical control* This can involve blocking or trapping insects ('glue' boards for whitefly), controlling temperature in green-houses, light traps, screens, metal barriers (to deter rodents), hand picking and so on.

(4) *Alternative chemical control (or better control over existing agro-chemicals)*

(i) The chemicals which control insect feeding and reproductive behaviour – pheromones – have been used successfully in experiments to control pests in agriculture and horticulture.

(ii) Better understanding of pest biology and ecology has led to a reduction of chemicals used. Examples include the application of lower doses of aphicides on cabbages to allow natural predators to survive and control remaining aphids.

(iii) Non-persistent insecticides on whitefly, followed by the introduction of predators, have solved the pest problems on some crops.

(iv) Knowledge of the economic threshold above which spraying is clearly a waste of money.

(v) Spraying at the right time to ensure the maximum medium- and long-term control of pests is assured.

(vi) Recognition that a high number of pests doesn't necessarily lead to damage (and vice-versa).

(vii) Proper placing and application of pesticides to kill pests and protect pest predators.

(viii) Recognition of when pest damage is merely cosmetic to a crop rather than physically and economically serious.

## Successful national and local IPM schemes

Several US examples of successful Integrated Pest Management are cited in the produce entries of this book. Additional examples are listed below.

(1) Good IPM means spraying chemicals only when you have to. So if we change perceptions of food quality we do not always have to spray. In the UK crops are regarded as clean if they grow without weeds and are not blemished. Others view clean crops as those not treated with or containing chemicals. The Royal Commission on Environmental Pollution attempted to discourage the spraying of crops simply to improve their cosmetic appearance rather than to prevent crop destruction by pests (HMSO 1979, pp68-72).

(2) Chinese agriculture has used integrated pest control based on studies of breeding insects, exclusion tactics and natural controls combined with the use of less dangerous pesticides. Fish and ducks for instance are used to control pests in rice paddy fields. China has 900 million people and is a major rice exporter growing 39% of the world's rice. She produces 100 agro-chemicals only and relies on just 7 organo-phosphorous insecticides, recognising that pesticides can be very hazardous to people (Van den Bosch, 1980, pp147-150).

(3) The entire sweet potato acreage in Cuba is under biological control. For peppers and corn, alternating planting dates reduced pesticide treatments from 28 to 12 in 1983. In the sugar crop, the sugar borer has been controlled by parasites since 1976/77. The citrus fruit blackfly is controlled biologically and the number of fungicide treatments on the crop has dropped from 15 to one or two treatments per year. On some farms, no insecticides have been applied for 4 years (Alexander and Anderson, 1984, pp31-41).

(4) Nicaragua has perhaps the best documented examples of IPM and the historical consequences, in the human and environmental health field, of high pesticide inputs. Swezey, Daxl and Murray provide a revealing and detailed analysis of pesticide use in Nicaragua and the short account below is drawn from their work (Swezey, Daxl and Murray, 1984, pp1-71).

Before the introduction of IPM, cotton production for export played a major part in Nicaraguan agriculture and led to a decline in the number of small food producers on the land and an increase in the use of insecticides to protect the cotton. The consequences of this were:

- cotton pests became resistant to pesticides.
- previously harmless and undetectable pests unknown in the 1940s and 1950s became important secondary pests.
- spray drift destroyed natural predators of pests not only on cotton but also corn and bean crops, and pests began to affect these crops.
- pesticide residues in people increased.
- between 1962 and 1972, 3,000 or more cases of acute pesticide poisoning occurred in agricultural workers (an annual rate of 176 per 1,000 population, eight times the US per capita rate).
- malaria incidence increased and in cotton-growing areas DDT became ineffective against the mosquito vector. Due to excessive agricultural spraying, resistance of the mosquito vector also occurred to organo-phosphorous, organo-chlorine and carbamate pesticides. The reported malaria cases in Nicaragua between 1972 and 1982 increased by over 400%.
- In 1977 a United Nations report estimated that insecticide-caused environmental and social damage cost $200 million a year in Nicaragua: foreign exchange from cotton exports totalled $141 million in 1973 (Falcon and Daxl, 1977).

The cost-benefit analysis clearly shows the economic and human health price paid by high and indiscriminate pesticide usage. Since the 1970s, some effective IPM schemes have been introduced and with them some of the problems attached to pesticide use have been reduced.

(5) Other examples of IPM include:

- in Cambridgeshire, England, experimental farms are using kestrels to control rodents which attack sugar beet and vegetable seed beds (*Farmers Weekly* 19 July 1985).
- in Cambridge University's Applied Biology Department, experimental inter-cropping of dwarf beans and cabbages, marigolds and vegetables, onions and carrots, beans and cauliflowers has greatly reduced crop losses from insects (*Farmers Weekly* 2 September 1983).
- in Malaysia, 40% of the oil palm and cocoa crops were lost until biological control by natural enemies was used.

• in the US, pests of corn, cotton, alfalfa, soybeans, grapes, citrus, walnut, tomatoes, apples and some vegetables have been effectively controlled by IPM and a minimum use of pesticides.

• in Britain, most greenhouse vegetable pests are controlled by IPM methods without the use of chemicals at all.

• in Marin County, California, the authorities reduced mosquito spraying by 90% through proper insect population monitoring, reduced pesticide use (by the simple expedient of not spraying mosquitoes in places never visited by people) and breeding-place management. At the same time the scheme achieved an overall reduction of the mosquito problem (Van den Bosch 1980, p155).

• in Thailand, successful IPM schemes have been mounted for soybeans and new schemes are mooted for rice, cotton and fruit trees (Napometh 1981, pp35-37).

Other examples of successful alternatives to the use of pesticides in food production in the developing countries come from cassava cultivation in Africa, soybeans in Brazil, bananas in Costa Rica, rice in South-East Asia and coconuts in the Pacific area (M. Hansen, *Escape from the Pesticides Treadmill*, IOCU, Penang, 1988).

## Auditing pesticides and their alternatives

The full social, economic, environmental and occupational health and safety consequences of using agri-chemicals across the world are little researched and little understood despite official protestations to the contrary. There is now an urgent need to carry out 'audits' on pesticides which go beyond narrow cost-benefit analyses, which often appear to concentrate on factors of profitability versus acute pesticide poisoning. These narrow analyses also frequently present data on the safe health and environmental effects of pesticides as complete or adequate for clearance when they are often incomplete and uncertain.

All too often assumptions are made that pesticides must be used because there is no alternative, because such pesticides are 'known' to be safe and because the profits and jobs created by their use far outweighs any adverse effects. These assumptions would be properly, openly and fully scrutinised by the audit method and would therefore probably ensure greater public confidence in revised pesticide approvals schemes.

Audits on the effects of pesticides reveal the economic as well as the social and environmental disadvantages (as well as advantages) of pesticide use, or of high and uncontrolled pesticide use – as in California and Oregon in the US, in Cuba, in Nicaragua and in parts of China.

## Audit concepts

No pesticides should be developed, marketed or used unless a full social, economic, environmental and occupational health and safety audit is made available by the manufacturers and scrutinised by competent staff in adequately funded and resourced government departments.

The audit should therefore examine the impact of a pesticide on jobs, communities, and the human and natural environment. It should look at the worst case as well as the best case analysis of pesticide use. It should look at and openly define and document the criteria used to describe 'acceptable' risks attached to pesticide use and 'acceptable' alternatives to such pesticides. The audit should also clearly note the uncertainties and data gaps on pesticide testing and use.

Such audits should be open to public comment – the 'scoping' of current US procedure – in the planning stages and made available to the public when complete. The audits would therefore involve manufacturers, importers, suppliers and, at a later stage, users and consumers. Users would include farmers, public authorities and local government. The nature and extent of the audit would therefore vary for each of these groups.

Direct *and* indirect costs of pesticide manufacture, use and disposal should be identified, with calculations of jobs created and jobs lost both by pesticide developments and by moves away from chemical farming.

The data requirements for approval in the UK under the Control of Pesticides Regulations 1986 do not mention auditing, nor do they touch on the social or, in a meaningful sense, the economic aspects of such an audit. There are references to the efficacy of pesticides but the data publicly available on the economic, social and environmental efficacy of pesticide use is very limited. There is therefore a pressing need for agreed and standard international auditing criteria.

The question of pollution caused by the manufacture and disposal of pesticides, the creation or loss of jobs by new pesticide developments, the energy and therefore further pollutions and job implications are all neglected. The job, food, pollution and health implications of using different pesticides, integrated pesticide management or organic methods are simply not part of current pesticide legislation.

In the UK the Food and Environment Protection Act itself does refer to 'the continuous development of means to protect the health of human beings, creatures and plants; to safeguard the environment and to secure safe, efficient and humane methods of controlling pests'. Auditing should form part of this development but it is ignored in the regulations. Auditing should be a key mechanism in operating the 'polluter pays' principle, for without an audit who will know who is polluting what, to what extent and how much they should pay?

## Audit topics

A. *Production costs and benefits*
   1. Raw materials extraction, energy, transport, water and air pollution.
   2. Processing. Energy, machinery costs, water and air pollution. Waste products disposal. Labour costs in development, etc.
   3. Costs of regulating, inspecting and prosecuting polluters.
   4. Jobs created/jobs lost through introduction of pesticides.
   5. Costs of unemployment of workers who lost jobs partly because of the greater 'efficiency' of pesticides over traditional methods.

B. *Distribution costs and benefits*
   1. Costs of sales, movement to suppliers – transport, storage, disposal.
   2. Costs of regulating, inspecting and prosecuting polluters.

C. *Usage costs and benefits*
   1. *Human.* Poisoning (accidental and deliberate), illnesses. Acute and chronic effects of active ingredients, inerts and

solvents. For operators, the public and through air, water and food pollution and contamination.

2. *Animal*. Mammals (pets and wildlife), birds, insects (loss of honey bees and effects on pollination), fish, invertebrates, soil fauna. Environmental: flora, pesticide effects on meadows, on farming practices and hence on soil erosion, soil state and impact on soil micro-organisms. Water and air pollution. Damage to other crops by spray drift, etc. Pest resistance. Damage to beneficial predators.

3. *Food production*. Implications of using pesticides, food chain contamination, pesticide residues.

4. Costs of regulating, inspecting and prosecuting polluters.

D. *Environmental protection and jobs*
   1. Jobs created in environmental safety, the prevention of pollution, and the control and rectification of past pesticide pollution.

E. *Costs and benefits of alternatives to high agro-chemical usage systems*
   1. Organic.
   2. Integrated Pest Management.

Audits will cover such issues as the polluter pays principle; food production and environmental and human survival; reversible and irreversible impacts; limits of the state of knowledge; local, regional, national and international implications and responses; and the viability of alternatives (IPM and organic production and the implications of these approaches in terms of food production, sustainability and environmental impacts).

Weaknesses of cost-benefit analysis include calculation of inputs, values, uncertainties, margins of error, and the problem of accepting science and economics as the most accurate and best guides to social and environmental policy-making given their inability to predict some risks.

## International comparisons

Pimentel in 1980 assessed that in the US 1 billion pounds by weight of pesticides were applied at the cost of $2.8 billion. Of this about 800 million pounds were applied to crops with an estimated benefit of $8.7 billion in reduced crop losses. The additional 200 million pounds of pesticides not used on crops produced benefits estimated at $2.2 billion. The grand total of benefits was $10.9 billion.

However, the indirect costs of pesticide usage in the US were estimated at $300 million for natural enemy losses, resistance and insurance costs plus $540 million to human and animal pesticide poisoning, honey bee poisoning, fishery and wildlife losses, and government pesticide pollution controls.

Direct costs of $2.8 billion plus indirect costs of $840 million gives a total cost of pesticide usage of $3.64 billion. Thus there was a return on pesticide investment of 3 dollars per dollar invested.

## Good models

1. California's Environment Quality Act requires that the cumulative impact of projects must be assessed by environmental impact reports. This should pick up mixing of pesticides with each other and with other chemicals in the environment.
2. The US National Environment Policy Act Regulations for implementation in 1978 opened the way for pesticide audits and involvement of community and environmental groups in the audit process at state and local level. (They are dealt with nationally by the Council on Environmental Quality based in the Executive Office of the US President).

# PART 2
# Guide to Foods

This section of the book lists a range of foods and drink which may be consumed by people in many countries. The lists of pesticides provided for each entry are not exhaustive nor are they all necessarily used or even approved in every country. However, as foods are now exported from one part of the world to another with great ease, it is quite possible that readers of this book may consume food produced many thousands of miles away with the use of pesticides not approved in their own country. For explanations of abbreviations, see Part 4.

## Classification of vegetables

The names of the vegetables and fruit cited are usually those common to the UK or the US. However, there are problems of definition and categorisation here. For instance, in England and Germany an endive is what the UK calls an endive but in France an endive is what the UK calls chicory. The US follows popular French definitions on endives (that it is chicory) but US scientific usage follows UK definitions on endives.

In the US the term 'collards' is quite common and refers to non-headed cabbages. These are all categorised under brassicas and cabbages in the following sections.

The term 'squash' for vegetables in the US is used as a general term to refer to squashes, pumpkins and marrows. The terms squashes and gourds may be used interchangeably there. In the UK marrows are not regarded as squashes and are usually categorised as cucurbits with courgettes and gherkins.

Calabrese is a type of broccoli. Raddichio is Italian red winter lettuce and is not connected to the radish.

Melons may be placed under three headings: muskmelon, cantaloupes and winter melons. In the US cantaloupes are often categorised separately from the other melon groups.

## The pesticide lists

The most acutely toxic pesticides listed in the produce section appear in the toxicity sections at the back of the book, where you will be able to find details of the effects of that chemical, where if at all it has been banned, and the basis for any regulatory action.

Other pesticides listed in Part 2 may not appear in Part 3. Their absence from the pesticide toxicity data does not mean that they are necessarily safe or dangerous. It does indicate the vast range of pesticides which may be applied to food crops, sometimes as often as 20 times or more in one season, and *the gaps in our knowledge about the effects of long-term low-level exposure of humans to pesticides*. Often there is no *evidence of absence* of the effects of pesticide on humans; rather, there is an *absence of evidence* of effects one way or another: a very different matter.

## Hazard assessments

Where national or international MRLs have been exceeded the entry will be marked**. This does not mean that all pesticides have been checked in all produce or that these are the only ones that present problems. Such a surveillance system would be impossible to operate. However, in some countries relatively small and unrepresentative samples of produce are checked for a relatively small number of pesticides. It is not therefore possible either to identify the risks or the consequences of exposure to pesticide residues in food in many countries and in many cases.

It is often stated that hazard = toxicity × exposure. Bear in mind when you look at the potential problem of pesticide residues in food that we still have a very poor picture of what precisely is the toxicity of long-term low-level exposure to pesticides which may mix with many other chemicals in our environment and be absorbed into humans who may be very young, very old, very ill or with very specialised diets. Bear in mind too that we cannot accurately measure our exposure to many pesticides or mixtures of pesticides in food, air and water.

## Gardeners

Some readers of this book may be gardeners who grow their own food. A list of common trade names for some of the pesticides referred to both here and in Part 3 appears in Part 4.

## Key sources of information for this section

Regional Agro-Pesticide Index (CIRAD/CNEARC), D. Jourdain and E. Hermout (ARSAP, Bangkok, Thailand): Vol 1 Asia (1989); Vol 2 Pacific (1990); Vol 3 Africa (1989).

North Carolina Agricultural Farm Chemicals Manual 1988 (North Carolina State University, Raleigh USA).

The UK Pesticide Guide edited by G. W. Ivens (CAB/BCPC, Exeter, 1990).

Pesticides 1989 (HMSO, London, 1989).

Pesticides Index, ed. Hamish Kidd and Douglas Hartley (CONRI and RSC, Nottingham, England, 1988).

The national reports on pesticide residues in food from government departments in the UK, US, Canada, Australia, Denmark, Norway, Sweden and Finland. Reports of the US NRC and the NRDC.

## Washing, peeling and cooking fruit and vegetables as a means of reducing residues

The most recent survey of the subject was published in London by *Which?* in October 1990.

**Washing** It is a good general rule of hygiene to wash fresh fruit and vegetables. To what extent washing will remove pesticide residues depends very much on the type or types of pesticide used, the fruit or vegetables involved and a number of other factors. For instance, washing apples and potatoes does not affect the levels of several common pesticide residues, even though such residues are mainly in or on the skin.

Contact pesticides are less likely to penetrate the skin of crops and are designed to work on contact with pests. Translocated or systemic weedkillers and insect killers are designed to work by entering plants and pests and so are generally not affected by washing. Pesticides used in post-harvest treatments are likely to leave greater quantities of residues from pesticides than those applied pre-harvest.

Washing with water is often as good a way of removing residues as specialist washes.

**Peeling**  Similar issues apply to peeling as to washing but generally peeling will be more effective because it will remove residues in the skin or on the surface. It will not remove most residues of systemic pesticides.

**Rubbing and scrubbing**  Rubbing may remove small amounts of surface residues. Scrubbing also removes residues if the scrubbing removes those parts of the surface which contain the residues.

**Trimming visible fat off meat and poultry**  This will remove low levels of some persistent pesticides which collect in animal fat.

**Discarding outer leaves**  This may remove higher residues from greenhouse sprays but will mean more of the fruit or vegetable may be lost.

**Cooking**  Cooking fruit and vegetables will often reduce pesticide residues further. However, in some instances, cooking may increase the quantities of certain pesticide residues or their metabolites. This has happened with pesticides used on tomatoes, apples and potatoes.

# A-Z OF FOODS

**Apples** In 1989, the average Briton consumed over 23½ lb of fresh apples. The figure for Americans is similar. Apples are exported from at least 40 different countries.

In the UK at least 86 different pesticide ingredients have been approved for use on or around apples. In 1989 MAFF reported that 37 out of 46 UK apple samples contained carbendazim and 24 out of 96 imported apples contained diphenylamine and 10 contained ethoxyquin. In 1983 a MAFF survey report estimated that 99.9% of dessert apples were treated with pesticides on average 26.8 times and very similar figures were recorded for cooking apples. 3 samples of UK cooking apples and 5 samples of dessert apples contained residues of metalaxyl above the CAC maximum residue level.\*\*

In a 1988/9 MAFF report it was revealed that of 6 samples of UK home-produced apple puree, one contained residues of carbendazim. Of 35 apple-based infant foods from retail outlets, 9 contained residues of carbendazim, 1 of metalaxyl, 1 of daminozide and 1 of UDMH. Of 57 samples of apple juice tested 16 contained carbendazim and 2 daminozide. Of 22 apple products tested in 1989 in the UK, 7 contained daminozide.

In the UK in 1988/9 only 24 samples of UK cooking apples were taken and tested for pesticide residues and only 27 pesticides sought. For dessert apples the figures were 23 UK samples, 39 foreign and 37 pesticides sought. In the cooking apples, residues of carbendazim, diphenylamine, metalaxyl, phosalone and vinclozolin were detected. In imported dessert apples, residues of azinphos-methyl, carbendazim, chlorpyrifos, dimethoate, diphenylamin, dithiocarbamates, phosalone and thiabendazole were detected. South African apples contained dimethoate, EBDCs and diphenylamine; New Zealand apples contained azinphos-methyl and chlorpyrifos; US apples contained azinphos-methyl, carbendazim and diphenylamine; French apples contained carbendazim, EBDCs, diphenylamine, phosalone and thiabendazole; and Spanish apples contained carbendazim and phosalone.

Australia in 1987 detected DDT, dicloran, endosulfan and chlorpyrifos in their apples. In 1986 the Danes detected azinphos-methyl, triazophos and methamidophos in imported apples.

In 1989 in 136 samples of domestic apples, Sweden detected endosulfan, carbendazim, diclofol, dimethoate and tetradifon. On imported apples the Swedes detected captan, folpet, carbendazim, chlorpyrifos, daminozide, diazinon, EBDCs, diphenylamine, phosalone, phosmet, thiabendazole and triazophos. Some French apples exceeded the Swedish MRLs on EBDCs,** carbendazim** and phosalone;** Italian apples did so on triazophos;** Argentinian apples on carbendazim** and Italian apples on diphenylamine.**

In 1988 62% of domestic US apples sampled contained pesticide residues but none over the US tolerance level. For imported fruit the figure was 55%.

43 different pesticides have been detected in apples. In Poland between 1986-88, residues of MBC and captan were detected but none over the Polish maximum residue levels. India in 1989 reported that residues detected in its apples in the past included DDT and BHC.

*Which?* magazine recommends that you wash and rub or peel apples, if your diet is already rich in fibre, to reduce residues. In the US the NRDC found that the following residues applied to apples could be washed off to some extent: captan, phosmet and azinphos-methyl. However, the effects of washing on diphenylamine and endosulfan were unknown.

**Known 'nasty' pesticides used on or around apples:** AMITROLE, AZINPHOS METHYL, BENOMYL, CAPTAN, CARBARYL, CYPERMETHRIN, DELTAMETHRIN, DICOFOL, DIMETHOATE, DINOCAP, DSM-S, GAMMA-HCH, MANCOZEB, NICOTINE, ODM, ZINEB.

**Other possibly hazardous pesticides used:** AMITRAZ, ASULAM, AZINPHOS-METHYL, BORDEAUX MIXTURE, BUPIRIMATE, CARBENDAZIM, 2-CHLOREOTHYLPHOSPHONIC ACID CHLORPYRIFOS, COPPER HYDROXIDE, COPPER SULPHATE, CUFRANEB, CYFLUTHRIN, DALAPON, 2, 4-DES, DICAMBA, DICHLOBENIL, DIFLUBENZURON, DITHIANON, DIURON, DODINE, FENITROTHION, FENVALERATE, FOSETYL-ALUMINIUM, GIBBERLINS, GLYPHOSATE, HEPTENOPHOS, ISOXABEN, MALATHION, MCPA, MECOPROP, MERCURIC OXIDE, METALAXYL, 1-NAPHTHYLACETIC ACID, OXADIAZON, PENCONAZOLE, PENDIMETHALIN, PENTANCHLOR, PERMETHRIN, PHORATE, PHOSALONE, PIRIMIPHOS-METHYL, PROPYZAMIDE, PYRAZOPHOS, PYRETHRINS, ROTENONE, SIMAZENE, SULPHUR, TAR OILS, TERBACIL, TETRADIFON, THIOPHANATE-METHYL, THIRAM, TRIADIMEFON, TRICHLORFON, TRICLOPYR, TRIFORINE, VINCLOZOLIN.

Apple pests can be controlled by the use of natural insect predators which must not be destroyed by harmful chemicals. In Russia the codling moth has been controlled by such predators. In California pheromone lure traps have been successfully used to catch codling moths so damaging to orchards of apple trees.

**Apricots** In the UK in 1988/9 only 12 imported samples of apricots were tested for residues and only 9 pesticides sought. Apricots from France, Spain, Greece, South Africa and Spain were found to contain dithiocarbomates but none above UK maximum residue levels.

In 1988/9 in Canada in an analysis of 71 imported apricots, acephate was detected in 1 sample, chlorpyrifos, carbaryl in 2, azinphos-methyl in 5, captan in 17, dichloran in 1, phosalone in 5, tetradifon in 1 of 45 samples tested.

In 1987 DDT, dicofol and endosulfan were found in dried apricots in Australia.

In 1989 Sweden tested 10 samples of apricots and found captan, folpet and chlorothalonil. Some Greek and Italian apricots exceeded Swedish MRLs for captan and folpet.**

In 1988 in the US 41% of domestic apricots sampled (49 in number) contained pesticide residues and 20% of the total sample violated US tolerance levels. The figure for apricots imported into the US containing pesticide residues was 71% (of a sample of 24) and none exceeded US tolerance levels.

**Known 'nasty' pesticides used on or around apricots:** AMITROLE, CHLOR-PYRIFOS, DIAZINON, DICOFOL, DSM (PROHIBITED FOR USE IN USSR AND RESTRICTED USE IN CALIFORNIA), ENDOSULFAN, MANCOZEB, OXYDEMETON-METHYL, THIOMETON, ZINEB.

**Other possibly hazardous pesticides used:** ASULAM, BORDEAUX MIXTURE, COPPER HYDROXIDE, COPPER SULPHATE, COPPER OXYCHLORIDE, DITHIANON, FENTHION, MALATHION, PROCHLORAZ, PROPICONAZOLE, TAR OILS, TETRADIFON, VINCLOZOLIN.

**Artichoke** In 1986 a MAFF survey found that 100% of a sample of UK artichokes had been treated with insecticides. Apparently very few artichokes have been tested for pesticide residues in the UK.

**Known 'nasty' pesticides used on or around artichokes:** AZINPHOS-METHYL, ENDOSULFAN, METHYL PARATHION, MEVINPHOS.

**Other possibly hazardous pesticides used:** METHIDATHION, PHOSALONE.

**Asparagus** Little testing has been done on asparagus outside the US and Sweden. In the UK in 1986 51.9% of a representative sample of asparagus was treated with insecticides; 17% with molluscicides; 29.8% with fungicides and 93.3% with herbicides.

In Sweden, no pesticide residues were found in 3 imported samples of asparagus.

In 1988 the US detained asparagus from one Chilean shipper because of pesticide residues. Of 96 imported asparagus sampled only 6% contained pesticide residues but 2% of these exceeded the US tolerance level.** The US National Research Council report on regulating pesticides found a small risk of oncogenicity from herbicides used on asparagus.

**Known 'nasty' pesticides used on or around asparagus:** CAPTAN, CARBOSULFAN (THAILAND), CYPERMETHRIN, DIURON, FONOFOS, LINDANE, LINURON, MANCOZEB, MANEB, METHOMYL, METHIOCARB (THAILAND), METHYL BROMIDE, NICOTINE, PARAQUAT, SIMAZINE, TRIAZOPHOS.

**Other possibly hazardous pesticides used:** CARBARYL, DALAPON, DIQUAT, 2, 4-DES, FLUAZIFOP, GLYPHOSATE, HEPTENOPHOS, IPRODIONE, MALATHION, MCPA, METALAXYL, NAPROPAMIDE, PERMETHRIN, SETHOXYDIM, SIMAZINE, SULPHUR, TERBACIL, THIABENDAZOLE.

**Aubergine** *(also known as eggplant or, in India, brinjal)* In 1988 the US detained aubergines from five different Dominican Republic shippers because of four different pesticide residues in the vegetable. Of 226 imported aubergines sampled in 1988 34% contained pesticide residues but under 1% were over the US tolerance level.** In the same year 53% of aubergines grown in the US contained pesticide residues but none over the approved levels.

Pesticides detected in aubergines in India include DDT and BHC.

**Known 'nasty' pesticides used on or around aubergines:** ACEPHATE (PACIFIC), CAPTAFOL (PACIFIC), CAPTAN, CARBARYL, CHLOROPICRIN, CYPERMETHRIN, DICOFOL, DIMETHOATE (PACIFIC), ENDOSULFAN, MANEB, NALED (PACIFIC), NICOTINE, ZINEB.

**Other possibly hazardous pesticides used:** COPPER SULPHATE (PACIFIC), ETHION (PACIFIC), FENBUTATIN OXIDE, FENVALERATE, HETENOPHOS, IPRODINE, MALATHION, METALAXYL, METHOMYL, METHOXYCHLOR, NALED, OXAMYL, PARATHION, PERMETHRIN, RESMETHRIN, SULPHUR, TRICHLORFON (PACIFIC), VINCLOZOLIN.

**Avocados** In 1989 Sweden tested 24 samples of imported avocados and found pesticide residues in none.

**Known 'nasty' pesticides used on or around avocados:** BENOMYL, CARBARYL, DIMETHOATE, DINOSEB, METHOMYL, METHYL BROMIDE, PARATHION, PARAQUAT.

**Other possibly hazardous pesticides used:** COPPER HYDROXIDE, 2, 4-D, DAZOMET, DIAZINON, FOSETYL-AL, GLYPHOSATE, MALATHION, METALAXYL, PIRIMIPHOS-METHYL, PRO-CHLORAZ, THIABENDAZOLE.

## Bamboo shoots
In the US in 1988, of 11 imported bamboo shoots sampled none contained pesticide residues.

## Bananas
In 1989, the average Briton consumed 13 lb of fresh bananas while the average American eats 11 lb. In the UK in 1988/9 63 samples of imported bananas were tested for 11 different pesticides. Carbendazim was identified in a Surinam sample, thiabendazole in a Colombian sample and permethrin in a sample of unknown origin.

In 1988 the US found residues of aldicarb in 2% of bananas sampled. The highest level detected was 0.12ppm when the US tolerance was 0.3ppm.

In Sweden in 1989 of 97 imported samples of bananas tested, 2 contained imazalil and 34 thiabendazole. In India in 1989 residues of DDT and BHC were reported in bananas.

Green bananas are immune to many pests and so crops harvested green should have been treated with fewer pesticides preharvest, but may be treated in some countries with pesticides to ripen them. Thick banana skins may also prevent several pesticides from being absorbed into the edible fruit.

**Known 'nasty' pesticides used on or around bananas:** ALDICARB, BENOMYL, CARBARYL, DICOFOL, DSM, DIURON, CARBENDAZIM, CARBOFURAN (ASIA), CHLORPYRIFOS, DIAZINON, LINURON, MANCOZEB, NALED (ASIA), PARAQUAT.

**Other possibly hazardous pesticides used:** ATRAZINE, 2,4-D, DALAPON, DICHLORVOS, GLYPHOSATE, IMAZALIL, ISOFENPHOS, MALATHION, MSMA, PERMETHRIN, PROPICONAZOLE, THIABENDAZOLE, TRIDEMORPH.

Banana pests include at least 6 species of lepidoptera. In Costa Rica an effective IPM scheme was introduced which required the ending of pesticide usage – as this had seriously affected the natural predators of the lepidoptera. When natural pest controls were allowed to re-emerge, they worked!

## Barley
In 1987 in England and Wales, samples of malted barley were analysed and of 136 tested in England, 82 contained

very low levels of organophosphorous pesticides (fenitrothion, chlorpyrifos-methyl and pirimiphos-methyl). In Scotland 60 out of 83 samples contained very low levels of chlorpyrifos-methyl and pirimiphos-methyl.

**Known 'nasty' pesticides used on or around barley:** AMITROLE, BENOMYL, BROMOXYNIL, CARBENDAZIM, CHLOROTHALONIL, CHLORPYRIFOS, CYPERMETHRIN, DE-LTAMETHRIN, DSM, EBDCS, FONOFOS, IOXYNIL, GAMMA-HCH, MANCOZEB, MANEB, OMETHO-ATE, OXYDEMETON-METHYL, PARAQUAT, TRIAZOPHOS, ZINEB.

**Other possibly hazardous pesticides used:** BENODANIL, CHLORMEQUAT, CLOPYRALID, CYANAZINE, 2,4-D, DALAPON, DICAMBA, DICHLOBENIL, ETHIRIMOL, FENITROTHION, FENPROPIMORPH, FERBAM, FLUTRIAFOL, GLYPHOSATE, IMAZALIL, IPRO-DIONE, ISOPROTURON, LINURON, MCPA, MECOPROP, METOXURON, PENDIMETHALIAN, PIRIMIPHOS-METHYL, PROPICONAZOLE, PROCHLORAZ, SIMAZINE, SULPHUR, TCA, TER-BUTRYN, THIABENDAZOLE, THIOPHANATE-METHYL, THIRAM, TRIADIMENOL, TRIDEMORPH, TRIFORINE.

# Beans

## Broad Beans and Green Beans In the UK in 1986, in a representative sample of broad beans, 91% had been treated with insecticides, 95.3% with seed treatments, 36% with fungicides and 86% with herbicides. In 1988/9 26 samples of broad bean crops were tested for residues of 4 pesticides (although many more pesticides are used on broad beans): no residues were found. Average UK consumption per person of fresh and frozen beans was 4.8 lb in 1989.

In Sweden in 1989 1 out of 9 samples of beans was found to contain omethoate residues. In 1989 Cyprus found some abnormal pesticide residue levels in its green beans. In 1988/9 Canada expressed concern about beans from Mexico and the US and monitored EBDC levels closely. In Poland between 1986-88, residues of dithiocarbamates were found on beans but not above Polish MRLs.

In the US in 1988 long beans from 9 Dominican Republic shippers were detained because of two pesticide residues, while green beans from 2 shippers from the Dominican Republic and one from Mexico were detained because of one pesticide residue.

In the US the average citizen eats 11 lb of green beans per year. The EPA approves 60 pesticides for use on green beans and the FDA can routinely detect only 60% of them. The NRC estimates a small risk of oncogenicity in humans from the pesticide residues found in US beans. The NRDC found that washing would reduce the residues of chlorothalonil which it found in US green beans, would not reduce methamidophos and acephate which it also found, and noted the effects of washing on dimethoate residues found was unknown.

**Known 'nasty' pesticides used on or around broad beans:** BENOMYL, CARBEN-DAZIM, CYPERMETHRIN, DIMETHOATE, DISULFOTON, DSM, PHORATE, TRIAZOPHOS.

**Other possibly hazardous pesticides used:** BENDIOCARB, DRAZOXOLON, FOSETYL-ALUMINIUM, HEPTENOPHOS, PIRIMICARB, THIABENDAZOLE, THIOMETON, THIRAM, VINCLOZOLIN.

Spray drift and other accidental contamination of bean crops means that a much wider list of pesticides than those cited here may end up on bean crops.

The Mexican bean beetle severely damaged bean crops in the Americas. The use of resistant varieties of bean helped to reduce that damage without using pesticides.

# French Beans
In the UK in 1986 53% of a representative sample of French beans were treated with insecticides, 80% with seed treatments, 87% with fungicides and 97% with herbicides.

**Known 'nasty' pesticides used on or around French beans:** ALDICARB, AZINPHOS-METHYL, CAPTAN, CARBARYL, CARBENDAZIM, DIMETHOATE, DSM, DSM SULPHONE, GAMMA-HCH, NICOTINE, THIRAM.

**Other possibly hazardous pesticides used:** AZIPROTRYNE, CARBETAMIDE, CAR-BOFURAN, CHLORPYRIFOS, CLOPYRALID, CHLORTHAL-DIMETHYL, CYANAZINE, DESMETRYN, DICLOFOP-METHYL, HEPTENOPHOS, MALATHION, PERMETHRIN, THIABENDAZOLE, TRIALLATE, TRIFLURALIN.

# Mung Beans
Of 20 samples of mung beans tested in the UK in 1986/7, 3 contained very low levels of endrin, quintozene and fenitrothion.

**Known 'nasty' pesticides used on or around mung beans:** ALACHLOR, ALDICARB, BENOMYL, CARBENDAZIM, CARBOFURAN, CARBOSULFAN, CHLORPYRIFOS, DI-AZINON, MANCOZEB, METHOMYL, MONOCROTOPHOS, OMETHOATE, OXYDEMETON-METHYL, PARAQUAT, PARATHION, TRIAZOPHOS.

**Other possibly hazardous pesticides used:** CHLORFLUAZURON, CYHALOTHRIN, FENPROPATHRIN, FLUAZIFOP-METHYL, ISOPROCARB, METHAMIDOPHOS, OXADIAZON, PHOS-ALONE, QUINALPHOS, THIODICARB.

# Runner Beans
In 1986 in a representative sample of UK runner beans, 66% had been treated with insecticides, 4% with

acaricides, 83% with seed treatments, 70% with herbicides and 13% with soil treatments. In 1988/9, 20 samples of runner beans were tested for residues of just 5 different pesticides; none was found.

**Known 'nasty' pesticides used on or around runner beans:** ALDICARB, AZINPHOS-METHYL, CAPTAN, CARBARYL, CARBENDAZIM, DIMETHOATE, DSM, DSM SULPHONE, GAMMA-HCH, NICOTINE, THIRAM.

**Other possibly hazardous pesticides used:** AZIPROTRYNE, CARBETAMIDE, CARBOFURAN, CHLORPYRIFOS, CLOPYRALID, CHLORTHAL-DIMETHYL, CYANAZINE, DESMETRYN, DICLOFOP-METHYL, HEPTENOPHOS, MALATHION, PERMETHRIN, THIABENDAZOLE, TRIALLATE, TRIFLURALIN.

## Soya Beans

In 1986 and 1987, 5 samples of soya beans were purchased from a UK retail outlet and tested for certain pesticide residues: 1 contained residues of gamma-HCH.

Inorganic bromides have been detected in soya bean grain and flour 60 days after harvest in India.

In the US in 1988, 43% of soya beans sampled contained pesticide residues but none above US regulatory standards.

**Known 'nasty' pesticides used on or around soya beans:** ALACHLOR, ALDICARB, CARBENDAZIM, CARBOFURAN, CYPERMETHRIN, DELTAMETHRIN, DIAZINON, ENDO-SULFAN, MANCOZEB, METHOMYL, MONOCROTOPHOS, PARAQUAT, PARATHION-METHYL, THIRAM, TRIAZOPHOS. Used on food or forage crops in the US: CARBARYL, METHYL PARATHION.

**Other possibly hazardous pesticides used:** BITERTANOL, CARBOXIN, DICHLOROPROPENE, ETHOPROP, FENAMIPHOS, FENITROTHION, FLUAZIFOP-BUTYL, LINURON, MALATHION, METALAXYL, METHAMIDOPHOS, OXADIOZON, PERMETHRIN, PHOSALONE, THIODICARB, TRIADIMEFON, TRIFLURALIN. Used on feed or forage crops in the US: ACEPHATE, CHLORPYRIFOS, FENVALERATE, METHOMYL, PERMETHRIN, THIODICARB.

In Brazil, integrated pest management rather than high chemical inputs have been used to control the caterpillars and bugs which prey on soya beans. Natural pests have proved effective controls.

## Other beans

In 1986 and 1987, 12 samples of lima beans were purchased from UK retail outlets and one contained pesticide residue in the tests on it. The residue found was gamma-HCH.

In the same period 4 samples of flageolet beans were tested; one contained gamma-HCH residues at very low levels. 5 samples of urd beans were tested and one contained very low levels of gamma-HCH.

Nine samples of adzuki beans, 2 of brown beans, 1 of moth beans, 2 of rice beans, 2 of rose-coco beans and 1 of white beans were also tested. None of these samples resulted in the detection of any organo-chlorine or organo-phosphorous pesticides.

**Known 'nasty' pesticides used:** CARBARYL, DICOFOL, DIMETHOATE, DISULFOTON, ENDOSULFAN, METHYL PARATHION, MEVINPHOS, PHORATE.

**Other possibly hazardous pesticides used:** ACEPHATE, DIAZINON, ESFENVALE-RATE, FENVALERATE, METHOMYL, METHOXYCHLOR, PARATHION, TRICHLORFON.

## Bean sprouts
In 1988 none of the domestic US bean sprouts tested for pesticide residues (11 in sample) contained any.

## Beef and dairy products
(see also **Milk; Goats**) In 1989, the average Briton consumed over 19½ lb of beef *and* veal, and 6½ lb of butter. In 1987, the average American consumed over 73 lb of beef and 15 lb of veal.

In 1988/9, of 7 UK-produced beef samples analysed, 2 contained dieldrin. Of 14 imported samples analysed, with 21 residues sought, 1 from Holland contained dieldrin, 1 unknown sample contained gamma-HCH. In 1988, of 18 samples of beef kidney fat, 1 contained heptachlor, 2 contained beta-HCH, 2 ppDDE and 2 dieldrin (19 different pesticide residues were sought).

In 22 samples of UK UHT cream tested in 1988/9, 2 contained gamma-HCH, 5 dieldrin, 2 ppDDE and 1 HCB. Figures for the same period for UK-produced yoghurts were: in 24 samples tested 2 contained HCB, 8 gamma-HCH, 1 dieldrin, 1 ppDDE. Of 9 yoghurt samples imported into the UK, 1 from Greece contained gamma-HCH and 1 ppDDE, 1 from West Germany contained ppDDE (32 pesticide residues were sought). Of 33 samples of UK retail dairy ice cream sampled in 1988/9, 5 contained gamma-HCH and 5 ppDDE (32 pesticide residues were sought). Of 14 samples of UK milk, by herd in 1988, 1 contained alpha-HCH, 2 beta-HCH, 6 gamma-HCH, 10 dieldrin and 4 ppDDE.

In the US only a small oncogenicity risk from pesticide residues in beef was identified, although beef was second highest in risk estimates on 15 foods and presented the greatest risk from herbicides. A 1989 report noted that some beef imported into the US contained heptachlor and chlordane.

In Canada in 1987/8 a small sample of imported cheese was tested for residues and contained aldrin/dieldrin, atrazine, azinphos-methyl, carbofuran, carbophenothion, chlorbromuron, chlordane, chlorbenzilate, chlorfenvinphos, chlorpyrifos, coumaphos, DDT, diazinon, dicofol, endosulfan, endrin, iprodione, lindane, permethrin, malathion, linuron, mevinphos, phosmet, tecnazene and vinclozolin. However, none were above the Canadian MRLs.

**Known 'nasty' pesticides used on or around cattle:** ALDRIN, DDT, CHLORDANE, DIAZINON, DICHLORVOS, ENDRIN, ETHION, CHLORPYRIFOS, HCH ISOMERS, HEPTACHLOR, MIREX, NALED, PHOSMET.

**Other possibly hazardous pesticides used:** AMITRAZ, BROMOPHOS, CHLORVFEN-VINPHOS, COUMAPHOS, CROTOXYPHOS, DIOXATHION, DURSBAN, FAMPHUR, FENTHION, FEN-VALERATE, FLUCYTHRINATE, MALATHION, METHOXYCHLOR, METHOPRENE, PERMETHRIN, PROPETAMPHOS, PYRETHRINS, RABON, TRICHLORFON.

Cattle may of course be exposed to a whole range of pesticides accidentally – in grass and other fodder crops treated with herbicides deliberately or through spray drift. Cattle in the UK have also been affected adversely by insecticides not used as veterinary products. For instance, in Kent, cattle have been sprayed with the insecticide phosalone and the fungicide iprodione by passing aircraft.

The effects of irradiation on beef containing pesticide residues have also not been fully researched.

**Beer** *(see also Hops; Cereals; Water)* In the UK, we drink a total of 10,368 million pints of beer each year (an average of just over half a pint a day for each adult and child). Under 5% is imported.

Beer contains hops, barley and water. Barley, in addition to being treated with pesticides before harvest may be treated with pesticides in storage after harvest. These could include malathion, pyrethrins, gamma-HCH, methyl bromide and ethylene dibromide in those countries who have not banned their use. Some breweries offer organic beer, some countries control pesticide use rigorously.

In the UK, Lincoln Green lager in 1989 became the first organic beer sold here. Other organic beers include Golden Promise bottled beer from the Caledonian Brewery Company in Edinburgh. Ross Brewing Company of Bristol in 1990 used organic barley for its beers.

**Beetroot** In the UK in 1986, 76% of a representative sample of beetroot was sprayed with insecticides, 95% with seed treatments, 2% with fungicides and over 97% with herbicides.

In 1988 in the US, 30% of a sample of imported red beets contained pesticide residues but none over US tolerance levels.

In 1987, dicloran and dicofol residues were found in canned beetroot in Australia. In 1989 no residues were found in either domestic or imported beetroot in Sweden.

**Known 'nasty' pesticide which may still be used on or around the produce in some countries:** DICOFOL.

**Other possibly hazardous pesticides used:** CHLORPROPHAM, CLOPYRALID, DICLORAN, ETHOFUMESATE, FENURON, MALATHION, METAMITRON, OXAMYL, PHENMEDIPHAM, PROPHAM, PYRAZOPHOS, PYRETHRINS, TRICHLORFON.

## Beet

**Known 'nasty' pesticides used on or around beet:** CARBARYL, MEVINPHOS, PARATHION.

**Other possibly hazardous pesticides used:** DIAZINON, METHOXYCHLOR, TRICHLORFON.

**Blueberries** In 1988 in the US 66% of domestic fruit sampled contained pesticide residues but none were over US tolerance levels.

**Known 'nasty' pesticides used on or around blueberries:** BENOMYL, CAPTAFOL.

**Other possibly hazardous pesticides used:** ASULAM, AZINPHOS-METHYL, CARBARYL, DICHLOBENIL, FLUAZIFOP, GLYPHOSATE, MALATHION, NAPROMIDE, NORFLURAZON, ORYZALIN, PARAQUAT, PRONAMIDE, SETHOXYDIM, SIMAZINE, TERBACIL, TRIFORINE.

**Bread** *(see also Wheat)* In 1989 the average Briton consumed almost 100 lb of bread.

In 1988 6% of UK bread samples tested contained more than one organophosphorous pesticide at low levels. In 1989 fewer than 3% of samples contained multiple residues. In 1988 residues were found in 32% of UK bread samples tested: in 1989 the figure was 22%.

In 1988 residues of methacrifos, pirimiphos-methyl, malathion, chlorpyrifos-methyl, etrimfos, fenitrothion, gamma-HCH, beta-HCH occurred in UK bread products but either no UK MRL existed for them or none of the samples exceeded the UK MRL. In 1989, pirimiphos-methyl, malathion, chlorpyrifos-methyl, etrimfos and gamma-HCH were again detected.

In 1989 pesticides were detected in UK bread but not above their reporting limits: these included aldrin, carbaryl, chlordane, chlorpyrifos-methyl, diazinon, dichlorvos, dieldrin, endosulfan, endrin, fenitrothion, alpha-HCH, beta-HCH, gamma-HCH, heptachlor, HCB, methacrifos, phosphamidon.

In the UK in 1989 James Erlichman of *The Guardian* reported that the Home Grown Cereals Authority had found pesticides were chemically hidden in grain and so impossible to detect, destroy or wash off. The greatest problem came with pesticides used to treat stored grain. Wholemeal flour contained twice the levels of residues as white flour and the highest levels of all came in bran.

In 1987 the following pesticides were detected in Australian bread (white or wholemeal): chlorpyrifos-methyl, fenitrothion, pirimiphos-methyl, permethrin. In 1987 the following residues were detected in Australian bran: chlorpyrifos-methyl, fenitrothion, pirimiphos-methyl, malathion, bioresmethrin.

**Broccoli** In 1986 in the US, 88% of a representative sample of broccoli and kale were treated with insecticides, 53% with seed treatments, 43% with fungicides and 94% with herbicides.

In 1989 in Sweden no residues were found in a sample of 5 domestic and 12 imported broccoli crops.

In 1988 in the US, of 122 imported broccoli plants sampled, 25% contained pesticide residues but none over the US tolerance levels. The US has 50 different pesticides registered with the EPA for use on broccoli and the FDA can routinely test for 70% of those. The NRDC detected a number of residues on crops and found that methamidophos and demeton could not be removed by washing while the effects of washing were unknown on DCPA, dimethoate and parathion.

**Known 'nasty' pesticides used on or around broccoli:** CARBARYL, CHLOROTHALONIL, CHLORPYRIFOS, DIMETHOATE, ENDOSULFAN, METHOMYL, MEVINPHOS, NALED, PARATHION, ZINEB.

**Other possibly hazardous pesticides used:** AZINPHOS-METHYL, DISULFOTON, ESFENVALERATE, FENVALERATE, IPRODIONE, METALAXYL, METHAMIDIPHOS, METHOXYCHLOR, PERMETHRIN, PHOSPHAMIDON, ROTENONE, SULPHUR.

## Brussels sprouts
In 1989 the average Briton consumed 3.3 lb of fresh brussels sprouts.

In the UK in 1986 in a representative sample, 99% of brussels sprouts were treated with insecticides, 24% with molluscicides, 22% with seed treatments, 61% with fungicides and 92% with herbicides.

In Sweden in 1989 EBDCs were found in 1 of a sample of 6 imported batches of brussels sprouts.

In 1988 in the US, 29% of imported brussels sprouts, from a sample of 51, were found to contain pesticide residues but none over the US tolerance level.

**Known 'nasty' pesticides used on or around brussels sprouts:** AZINPHOS-METHYL, CARBARYL, CARBENDAZIM, CHLOROTHALONIL, DIMETHOATE, ENDOSULFAN, MANEB, METHOMYL, METHYL-PARATHION, MEVINPHOS, NALED, PARATHION, ZINEB.

**Other possibly hazardous pesticides used:** CHLORPYRIFOS, DIAZINON, DISULFOTON, ESFENVALERATE, FENVALERATE, METHAMIDOPHOS, METHOXYCHLOR, METALAXYL, PERMETHRIN, ROTENONE, PCNB, TRICHLORFON.

## Cabbages
The average Briton eats over 10 lb of fresh cabbage a year. The average American eats about 5 lb.

In the UK in 1988 the following percentages of cabbages in a representative sample were treated with pesticides:

| Type | insecticides | fungicides | herbicides | seed treatments |
|---|---|---|---|---|
| savoy | 99% | 44% | 51% | 9% |
| autumn/summer | 95% | 27% | 85% | 25% |
| spring | 47% | 10% | 62% | 41% |
| white | 96% | 39% | 88% | 17% |
| winter | 89% | 41% | 80% | 46% |

In 1988/9, 39 UK and 8 imported samples of green cabbage were tested for 19 different pesticide residues and none were found.

In India in 1989, residues of DDT and lindane were reported in cabbages. In Poland between 1986-88, residues of diazinon, dimethoate, lindane and other organochlorine pesticides were recorded but none over the Polish MRLs.

The NRC estimates a low risk of oncogenicity from herbicides used on cabbages. In 1988 in the US, 11% of 37 imported cabbages contained pesticide residues but none exceeded the US tolerances. The NRDC found a range of pesticides in cabbage of which permethrin could be washed off, methamidophos could not and the effects of washing on dimethoate, fenvalerate and BHC were unknown.

**Known 'nasty' pesticides used on or around cabbages:** AZINPHOS-METHYL, CARBARYL, CARBENDAZIM, CHLOROTHALONIL, CYPERMETHRIN (ASIA), DELTAMETHRIN (ASIA), DIMETHOATE, ENDOSULFAN, MANEB, METHOMYL, METHYL-PARATHION, MEVINPHOS, NALED, PARATHION, ZINEB.

**Other possibly hazardous pesticides used:** ABAMECTIN (ASIA), CHLORPYRIFOS, CHLORFLUAZURON (ASIA), CYFLUTHRIN (ASIA), DIAZINON, DISULFOTON, DIFLUBENZURON (ASIA), ESFENVALERATE, FENVALERATE, FLUFENOXURON (ASIA), MALATHION (ASIA), METH-AMIDOPHOS, METHOXYCHLOR, METALAXYL, PERMETHRIN, PIRMICARB (ASIA), PROTHIOFOS (ASIA), ROTENONE, PCNB, TRICHLORFON.

Cabbage pests can be controlled by a variety of non-chemical means. In the USSR various pests are controlled by the use of potted flowering plants, one to every 400 cabbages, which promote predators of cabbage pests and so ensure effective biological controls.

Various cabbage pests are also deterred by the use of kale as a trap crop. The pests go on the kale and then can be destroyed easily, or will do much less damage to the cabbage.

Potato leafhopper attacks on cabbages can also be reduced by growing pest-resistant varieties of cabbage.

## Chinese cabbage
In the UK in 1986, in a representative sample of chinese cabbage, 100% of the crop were treated with insecticides, 26% with seed treatments, 62% with fungicides, 99% with herbicides. In 1988/9, samples of 13 UK and 10 imported cabbages were tested for 21 pesticide residues; in the UK samples, 9 contained inorganic bromides; of the imports, 9 contained inorganic bromides, 2 pirmicarb (from Italy and Netherlands).

In Sweden in 1989, 3 of 58 samples of imported chinese cabbage contained inorganic bromides and 1 from Spain was over the Swedish MRL for EBDCs.**

In 1988 in the US, 67% of a sample of 36 chinese cabbage contained pesticide residues.

**Known 'nasty' pesticide used on or around chinese cabbage:** EBDCS.

**Other possibly hazardous pesticide used:** PIRMICARB.

## Calabrese
In the UK in 1986, in a representative sample of UK calabrese, 41% were treated with seed treatments, 13% with fungicides and 91% with herbicides.

**Known 'nasty' pesticides used on or around calabrese:** AZINPHOS-METHYL, CARBARYL, CARBENDAZIM, CHLOROTHALONIL, DIMETHOATE, ENDOSULFAN, MANEB, METH-OMYL, METHYL-PARATHION, MEVINPHOS, NALED, PARATHION, ZINEB.

**Other possibly hazardous pesticides:** CHLORPYRIFOS, DIAZINON, DISULFOTON, ESFENVALERATE, FENVALERATE, METHAMIDOPHOS, METHOXYCHLOR, METALAXYL, PER-METHRIN, ROTENONE, PCNB, TRICHLORFON.

## Cantaloupes _(see Melons)_
A commonly used American term which does not include water melons or honeydew melons.

## Carrots
The average Briton eats over 13 lb of carrots a year. The average American eats 8 lb.

In 1986 in a representative sample of UK carrots, 92% were sprayed with insecticides, 54% with seed treatments, 28% with fungicides and 94% with herbicides.

In 1988 in the US, 41% of a sample of 83 imported carrots contained pesticide resudues and 1% of the sample exceeded US tolerance levels.** The NRDC detected several residues in US carrots of which DDT could be washed off, trifluralin could not and the effects of washing on parathion, diazinon and dieldrin were unknown.

In 1989 in Sweden, 2 of 57 imported carrot samples contained bromophos, 2 chlorfenvinphos and 1 diazinon. In Poland in the late 1980s, residues of diazinon, linuron, HCB, DDT, lindane and prometrin were all detected but only lindane** exceeded the Polish MRLs. Canadians in 1986 detected 1% of their domestic carrot crop exceeding the MRL on linuron.** In Australia in 1987 DDT and dicloran were found in carrots.

**Known 'nasty' pesticides used on or around carrots:** ALDICARB, BENOMYL, CAPTAN, CARBARYL, CHLOROTHALONIL, DIMETHOATE, DISULFOTON, DSM, MANEB, MAN-COZEB, OXYDEMETON-METHYL, PHORATE, THIRAM, TRIAZOPHOS, ZINEB.

**Other possibly hazardous pesticides used:** ALLOXYDIM-SODIUM, BROMOPHOS, CHLORPROPHAM, CHLORFENVINPHOS, COPPER HYDROXIDE, DALAPON, DCN, DI-1-P-METHANE, DIAZINON, DICLOFOP-METHYL, FENURON, FLUAZIFOP-METHYL, IPRODINE, LINURON, MALATHION, METALAXYL, METOXURON, MITC, PENTACHLOR, PIRIMICARB,

PIRIMIPHOS-METHYL, PROMETRYN, PYRAZOPHOS, QUINALPHOS, SETHOXYDIM, TCA, THIA-BENDAZOLE, TRIADIMEFON, TRIALLATE, TRIPHENYLTIN HYDROXIDE.

Commercial growers and gardeners have been able to reduce or even cease the use of pesticides to control carrot fly by inter-cropping onions in the carrot crop. This deters the carrot fly.

**Cauliflower** The average Briton eats about $7^1/_2$ lb of cauliflower a year.

In 1986, in a representative sample of UK cauliflowers, 87% were treated with insecticides, 6% with pesticide seed treatments, 23% with fungicides and 77% with herbicides. In 1988/9 in the UK 38 domestically produced samples and 13 imported samples of cauliflower were tested for 19 different residues; none were found.

In 1988 in the US, 11% of 54 imported cauliflowers contained pesticide resudues but none over the US tolerance level. The NRDC found chlorothalonil, dimethoate, diazinon, endosulfan and methamidophos in US cauliflowers but washing was known to reduce residues of only the first of these chemicals on vegetables.

In India in 1989 it was reported that residues of DDT, BHC, lindane, heptachlor and aldrin/dieldrin had been detected in domestic produce. In Poland in 1986-88, propoxur, dimethoate, DDT, lindane and other HCH isomers were detected but none above Polish MRLs.

**Known 'nasty' pesticides used on or around cauliflowers:** AZINPHOS-METHYL, CARBARYL, CARBENDAZIM, CHLOROTHALONIL, DIMETHOATE, ENDOSULFAN, MANEB, METH-OMYL, METHYL-PARATHION, MEVINPHOS, NALED, PARATHION, ZINEB.

**Other possibly hazardous pesticides used:** CHLORPYRIFOS, DIAZINON, DIS-ULFOTON, ESFENVALERATE, FENVALERATE, METHAMIDOPHOS, METHOXYCHLOR, METAL-AXYL, PERMETHRIN, ROTENONE, PCNB, TRICHLORFON.

**Celeriac** In the UK in 1986 100% of a representative sample of celeriac received pesticide seed treatment.

**Known 'nasty' pesticides used on or around celeriac:** CHLOROTHALONIL, DSM, NICOTINE.

**Other possibly hazardous pesticides used:** CHLORPROPHAM, QUINALPHOS, PEN-TANOCHLOR, PYRAZOPHOS, TRIFLURALIN.

**Celery** In 1986 in the UK, in a representative sample of domestic celery, 85% were treated with insecticides, 23% with seed treatments, 94% with fungicides, 100% with herbicides, 20% with growth regulators.

In 1988 in the US, 74% of 35 imported celery plants contained pesticide residues but none over the US tolerance level. In the US the EPA has approximately 60 pesticides registered for use on celery and the FDA can routinely detect just 50% of those as residues. The NRDC found that dicloran and chlorothalonil could be washed off but acephate and methamidophos could not and the effects of washing on endosulfan were unknown. Trimming leaves and tops of celery might reduce residues of chemicals like methomyl.

In Australia in 1987 permethrin was detected on celery. In Canada in 1988/9 concern was expressed about celery from Mexico and the US: with acephate, ethion, chlordimeform, permethrin and methamidophos monitored for in celery imports. In Poland between 1986 and 1988 diazinon, linuron and dimethoate were all detected on Polish celery but none above Polish MRLs.

In Sweden in 1989, of 27 celery batches sampled, 5 contained chlorothalonil, 1 bromophos-ethyl, 1 methamidophos, and 1 parathion. Some Spanish, Italian and US celery exceeded Swedish MRLs on chlorothalonil,** as did Israeli celery on methamidophos** and Dutch celery on chlorothalonil.**

**Known 'nasty' pesticides used on or around celery:** BENOMYL, CAPTAN, CARBENDAZIM, CHLOROTHALONIL, CYPERMETHRIN, DIMETHOATE, DISULFOTON, DSM, MANEB, MANCOZEB, NICOTINE, ODM, PHORATE, TRIAZOPHOS, ZINEB.

**Other possibly hazardous pesticides used:** ANILAZINE, BORDEAUX MIXTURE, BROMOPHOS, CHLORFENVINPHOS, CHLORPROPHAM, COPPER HYDROXIDE, COPPER OXYCHLORIDE, CUPRIC AMMONIUM CARBONATE, DIAZINON, DICLOFOP-METHYL, FERBAM, GIBBERLLINS, HEPTENOPHOS, LINURON, MALATHION, METIRAM, PENTANCHLOR, PERMETHRIN, PIRIMICARB, PROPAMCARB HYDROCHLORIDE, PROMETRYN, QUINALPHOS, THIABENDAZOLE, THIOPHANATE METHYL, VINCLOZOLIN.

**Cereals** (see also Bread; Wheat; Oats) In 1989, each person in the UK consumed on average over 173 lb of cereals of all sorts. In 1988 the average Briton consumed $14^1/_2$ lb of breakfast cereals.

In 1987 permethrin was detected in infant cereals in Australia.

In the UK between 1985 and 1986, 107 samples of rye products were tested and 19 contained residues of pesticides. These included etrimfos and pirimiphos-methyl, both at very low levels.

**Cheese** *(see also Beef and dairy products; Sheep)* In 1989, each person in the UK consumed on average over 12 lb of natural cheese. In 1987, each American consumed on average over 24 lb of cheese – excluding cottage cheese.

In 1988 in the US, 124 samples of domestic cheese and cheese products were tested for pesticides; residues were found in 17%; in 2%, US regulatory controls were breached.**

Between 1984 and 1987, samples of Scottish and imported cheese were analysed for pesticide residues in the UK. In 1984, 20 out of 20 Scottish samples contained residues which included HCB, isomers of HCH including gamma-HCH and dieldrin. Between 1986 and 1987, 86 of 177 UK-produced cheese samples contained residues. These included HCH isomers and dieldrin. 53 of 161 imported cheese samples in the UK between 1986 and 1987 contained residues – including HCH isomers and dieldrin.

**Cherries** *Which?* magazine in 1990 recommended washing cherries and shaking in water to reduce residues.

In 1988 50% of domestic US cherries sampled (101 in sample) contained pesticide residues but only 1% violated US tolerance levels.** For imported cherries the figures were 61% and 0%. The NRDC recommended washing to remove malathion, dicloran and captan but noted that the effects of washing on parathion and diazinon also detected on US cherries was unknown.

In Sweden in 1989, of 25 imported cherry samples, 1 contained endosulfan, 2 dicloran, 4 omethoate and 1 parathion. In Poland between 1986 and 1988, cypermethrin was detected on cherries but not above the Polish MRL.

**Known 'nasty' pesticides used on or around cherries:** AMINOTRIAZOLE, AZINPHOS-METHYL, CARBENDAZIM, CYPERMETHRIN, DELTAMETHRIN, DIMETHOATE, DSM, DSM-S, ODM.

**Other possibly hazardous pesticides used:** ASULAM, BENODANIL, BORDEAUX MIXTURE, CHLORPYRIFOS, CLOFENTEZINE, COPPER HYDROXIDE, COPPER OXYCHLORIDE, COPPER SULPHATE, CYFLUTHRIN, 2, 4-DES, FENITROTHION, GLYPHOSATE, ISOXABEN, MALATHION, OCTHILINE, OMETHOATE, PENDIMETHALIN, PENTACHLOR, PHOSALONE, PIRIMICARB, PIRIMIPHOS-METHYL, PROPYZAMIDE, PYRETHRINS, SIMAZINE, SODIUM MONOCHLOROACETATE, TAR OILS, TETRADIFON, VINCLOZOLIN.

**Chicken** *(see Fowl; Poultry)*

**Chickpeas** *(see Peas)*

**Chicory** In the UK in a representative sample of chicory crops, 50% of the crops received pesticide seed treatments and 50% received herbicide treatments.

In Sweden in 1989 1 imported load of chicory leaves contained iprodione residues.

**Known 'nasty' pesticides used on or around chicory:** CYPERMETHRIN, NICOTINE.

**Other possibly hazardous pesticides used:** HEPTENOPHOS, PROPYZAMIDE, QUINTOZENE.

**Chilli peppers** In California in 1986 S,S,S-Tributyl-phosphorotrithioate (DEF), an organo-phosphorous pesticide registered for use only on cotton, was found on chilli peppers and other food crops. DEF had extensive toxicological data gaps and had not therefore been fully evaluated. No action level existed for it in food. Again this illustrates the need for extensive and thorough monitoring and enforcement of pesticide regulations.

In Sweden in 1989 1 sample of chilli peppers contained dichlorvos.

**A possibly hazardous pesticide used on or around chilli peppers:** DICHLORVOS.

**Chocolate** (see Cocoa)

**Cocoa** In 1989, each person in the UK consumed on average almost $1/2$ lb of cocoa and drinking chocolate.

BHC residues have been detected in cocoa.

**Known 'nasty' pesticides used on or around cocoa plants:** ACEPHATE, ALDRIN, BENOMYL, CARBARYL, CHLORDANE, DEMETON METHYL, DIAZINON, DICHLORVOS, DICROTOPHOS, DIURON, ENDOSULFAN, LINDANE, MANCOZEB, METHYL BROMIDE, NALED, PARAQUAT, PHOSPHINE, 2, 4, 5-T.

**Other possibly hazardous pesticides used:** AMETRYN, ATRAZINE, COPPER HYDROXIDE, CUPROUS OXIDE, 2,4-D, DALAPON, FENITROTHION, FENTHION, FLUAZIFOP-BUTYL, GLYPHOSATE, METALAXYL, METRIBUZIN, PERMETHRIN, PICLORAM, PROPOXUR, SIMAZINE, TRICHLORFON.

**Coconuts** In the UK in 1988/9, of 5 samples of coconut analysed, 1 contained residues of gamma-HCH (lindane) and 5 contained residues of inorganic bromides.

In 1988 in the US no imported coconuts, from a sample of 14, contained any pesticide residues.

**Known 'nasty' pesticides used on or around coconuts:** AMITROLE, CARBARYL, CHLORDANE, CHLORPYRIFOS, CREOSOTE, DDT, DIAZINON, DIURON, LINDANE, MONO-CROTOPHOS, PARAQUAT, 2, 4, 5-T.

**Other possibly hazardous pesticides used:** ATRAZINE, DALAPON, DIQUAT, FENITROTHION, GLYPHOSATE, IMAZAPYR, MALATHION, MCPA, METRIBUZIN, MSMA.

Alternatives to chemical pest control have been effective on coconut crops. The coconut moth was successfully controlled in Fiji by a parasitic fly.

**Coffee** In 1989, each person in the UK consumed on average almost $1/2$ lb of bean and ground coffee and over $1^1/2$ lb of instant coffee. In 1987, each American consumed on average over $7^1/2$ lb of coffee.

In the US in 1989 it was reported that heptachlor/chlordane residues had been found in imported coffee.

**Known 'nasty' pesticides used on or around coffee:** ACEPHATE, BENOMYL, CAPTAN, CARBARYL, CARBOFURAN, CHLORDANE, DIAZINON, DICROTOPHOS, DIMETHOATE, DIURON, ENDOSULFAN, MANCOZEB, MONOCROTOPHOS, OXYCARBOXIN, PARAQUAT, PARA-THION, PICLORAM, ZINEB.

**Other possibly hazardous pesticides used:** AMETRYN, COPPER OXYCHLORIDE, CUFRANEB, FENTHION, GLYPHOSATE, MALATHION, METRIBUZIN, PERMETHRIN, PRO-PICONAZOLE, TRIADIMEFON.

It is generally accepted that beverages are not an important source of pesticide residues in our diet.

Coffee pests can be effectively controlled by non-chemical means. The autestin bugs or thrips can be controlled by pruning, which creates a mulch near the plant which in turn provides conditions suitable for parasites of this coffee bug.

**Coriander** In 1988 the US detained coriander from all Mexi-can shippers because of five different pesticide residues in the spice. In the same year 17% of imported coriander contained pesticide residues from a sample of 65.

**Corn** *(also known as Maize)* Each year the average American eats 11 lb of corn. In 1988 in the US only 2% of domestically grown corn, from a sample of 123, contained pesticide residues and none exceeded the US tolerance level. For imported corn into the US, 100% of the sample of 42 was free of pesticide residues. Eight different pesticides have been detected in US corn. The

NRDC noted that carbaryl found in the corn could be reduced by washing but that sulfallate, chlorpyrifos, dieldrin and aldrin, also detected, were unknown quantities in terms of washing off residues.

In Canada in 1987/8, 1% of domestic corn sampled contained glyphosate and 9% glyphosate metabolites, but none over Canadian MRLs.

**Known 'nasty' pesticides used on or around corn:** On corn as field and forage crops in the US: CARBARYL, CARBOFURAN, DISULFOTON, DIMETHOATE, FONOFOS, METHYL PARATHION, PHORATE.

**Other possibly hazardous pesticides used:** CARBOFURAN, ETHOPROP, TERBUFOS. On corn as field or forage crops in the US: CHLORPYRIFOS, FENVALERATE, MALATHION, METHOMYL, PERMETHRIN, TRICHLORFON, TERBUFOS.

## Courgettes (also known as Cucurbits) In the UK in 1986 75.8% of a representative sample of courgettes received insecticide treatments, 20.5% received seed treatments, 61.7% were treated with fungicides and 38.1% with herbicides.

**Known 'nasty' pesticides used on or around courgettes:** CYPERMETHRIN, DIMETHOATE, DSM, DISULFOTON, MANEB, NICOTINE, TRIAZOPHOS, ZINEB.

**Other possibly hazardous pesticides used:** BENDIOCARB, BUPIRIMATE, DIPHENAMID, HEPTENOPHOS, IMAZALIL, IPRODIONE, OXAMYL, PIRIMICARB, PROPAMOCARB HYDROCHLORIDE, PYRAZOPHOS, THIABENDAZOLE, THIRAM.

## Cranberry In 1988 in the US no fruit sampled for pesticide residues contained any.

**Pesticide which may be used on or around cranberries:** ASULAM.

## Cucumber The average Briton eats nearly 4 lb of fresh cucumber a year.

In 1988 in the US 61% of a sample of domestic cucumbers contained pesticide residues but none were over the tolerance level. 63% of a sample of 256 imported cucumbers contained pesticide residues. In 1988 the US detained one Canadian shipper's cucumbers because of pesticide residues. The EPA has 75 pesticides registered for use on cucumbers and the FDA routinely can identify only approximately 60% of them. Of residues identified in USA crops – dieldrin, endosulfan, methamidophos, dimethoate, chlorpyrifos – none could apparently be washed off.

In 1988/9 in Canada residues of chlorothalonil, diazinon, dicofol-p, aldrin, dieldrin, carbofuran, heptachlor, iprodione and endosulfan were identified in domestic produce.

In Sweden in 1989, of 144 domestic cucumbers sampled, 1 contained endosulfan and 6 mevinphos (1 over the MRL);** of 137 imported samples, 6 contained aldrin/dieldrin, 2 captan/folpet, 1 chlorothalonil, 5 endosulfan, 2 acephate, 2 EBDCs, 8 methamidophos, 2 trichlorfon. In a Swedish test on imported dill cucumbers, 1 of 5 contained chlorpyrifos. In the samples some Spanish cucumbers exceeded Swedish MRLs on mevinphos.**

In Poland between 1986-88 residues of EBDCs, MBC and metalaxyl were detected in Polish cucumbers but none above the Polish MRLs. In Cyprus in 1989, abnormal levels of residues were detected in some cucumbers.

**Known 'nasty' pesticides used on or around cucumbers:** AZINPHOS-METHYL, BENOMYL, CARBARYL, CARBENDAZIM, CHLOROTHALONIL, CYPERMETHRIN, DELTAMETHRIN, DIAZINON, DICOFOL, DINOCAP, DICHLORVOS, DSM, ENDOSULFAN, FOLPET, GAMMA-HCH, METHOMYL, NALED, NICOTINE, THIRAM, ZINEB.

**Other possibly hazardous pesticides used:** BUPIRIMATE, COPPER OXYCHLORIDE, CUPRIC AMMONIUM CARBONATE, DICLORAN, ESFENVALERATE, ETRIDIAZOLE, FENARIMOL, FENBUTATIN OXIDE, FENVALERATE, HEPTENPHOS, IMAZALIL, IPRODIONE, METHOXYCHLOR, MEVINPHOS, PARATHION, PERMETHRIN, PETROLEUM OILS, PHOSPHAMIDON, PIRIMICARB, PROPAMOCARB, PROPOXUR, PYRETHRINS, QUINTOZENE, SULPHUR, TETRADIFON, TRIADIMEFON, TRIFORINE.

In the US the pickleworm pest of pickling cucumbers has been controlled simply by growing crops in the spring before the worm invades from the Gulf coast. This method does not require expensive chemicals to work.

## Cucurbits *(see Courgettes)*

**Currants** *(Red and Black Currants; for dried fruits see **Grapes**)* In Poland in 1986-88 residues of EBDCs were found in currants but not above Polish MRLs. Danes found pyrazophos** in some of their red currants above Danish MRLs in 1986; likewise captafol** and pyrazophos** above Danish MRLs in 1986 and, in 1987, black currants exceeded Danish MRLs on pyrazophos.**

In Sweden some Swedish currants exceeded Swedish MRLs on endosulfan.**

**Known 'nasty' pesticides which may be used on or around currants:** AZINPHOS-METHYL, BENOMYL, CARBARYL, CARBENDAZIM, CHLOROTHALONIL, CYPER-METHRIN, DIMETHOATE, DINOCAP, DSM, DSM-S, DIURON, ENDOSULFAN, MANOZEB, MANEB, ODM, PARAQUAT, ZINEB.

**Other possibly hazardous pesticides used:** ASULAM, BORDEAUX MIXTURE, BUPIRI-MATE, CRESYLIC ACID, CHLORPROPHAM, CHLORPYRIFOS, CHLORTHAL-DIMETHYL, COPPER HYDROXIDE, COPPER SULPHATE, CUFRANEB, CUPRIC AMMONIUM CARBONATE, CYFLUTHRIN, DALAPON, 2,4-DES, DICHLOBENIL, DICHLOFLUANID, DIFLUBENZURON, DODINE, FENARIMOL, FLUAZIFOP-METHYL, FENITROTHION, HEPTENOPHOS, ISOXABEN, LENACIL, MCPB, METH-IOCARB, NAPROPAMIDE, OXADIAZON, PENDIMETHALIN, PENTACHLOR, PIRIMICARB, PRO-PYZAMIDE, SIMAZINE, SODIUM MONOCHLOROACETATE, SULPHUR, TAR OILS, TETRADIFON, TRIADIMEFON, TRICHLORFON, VINCLOZOLIN.

Pests of black currants have been successfully controlled by 'roguing' – the removal and destruction of infected bushes – which is especially effective against the black currant gallmite. This method removes the need to use pesticides.

## Damsons

**Known 'nasty' pesticides used on or around damsons:** AMINOTRIAZOLE, AZINPHOS-METHYL, CYPERMETHRIN, DELTAMETHRIN, DSM, DSM-S, CARBENDAZIM, O-DM.

**Other possibly hazardous pesticides used:** ASULAM, BENODANIL, BORDEAUX MIXTURE, CHLORPYRIFOS, CLOFENTEZINE, COPPER OXYCHLORIDE, COPPER SULPHATE, CUFRANEB, CYFLUTHRIN, 2,4-DES, DIFLUBENZURON, DIMETHOATE, FENITROTHION, GLYPHO-SATE, ISOXABEN, MALATHION, NAPROMIDE, 1-NAPHTHYLACETIC ACID, OCTHILINONE, OMETHOATE, PENDIMETHALIN, PENTACHLOR, PHOSALONE, PIRIMICARB, PIRIMIPHOS-METHYL, PROPYZAMIDE, PYRETHRINS, SODIUM MONOCHLOROACETATE, SIMAZINE, TAR OILS, TETRADIFON, VINCOZOLIN.

**Dates** In the UK in 1988/9, 9 samples of imported fresh dates were taken and 6 different pesticide residues sought. 1 residue of malathion was detected in US dates. No residues were detected in Egyptian or Israeli dates at reportable levels.

**Known 'nasty' pesticides used on or around dates:** CYPERMETHRIN, DDT, DELTAMETHRIN, DIELDRIN, GAMMA-HCH.

**Other possibly hazardous pesticides used:** ETHION, FENPROPIMORPH, FERBAM, MALATHION, PHOSALONE, PIRIMIPHOS-METHYL, SULPHUR.

**Deer** *(see Venison)*

**Eggs** *(see Fowl; Poultry)*

**Endives** In 1988 the US detained one Canadian and one Italian shipper's cargo of endives because of pesticide residues. In the same year in the US 23% of a sample of 93 imported endive/chicory plants contained pesticide residues.

**Known 'nasty' pesticides used on or around endives:** CYPERMETHRIN, MANEB, NICOTINE, ZINEB.

**Other possibly hazardous pesticides used:** HEPTENOPHOS, QUINTOZENE, PROPYZAMIDE.

**Figs** In the UK in 1986/7, 12 samples of dried figs from Egypt and Greece were analysed and all 12 contained inorganic bromides. Sweden in 1989 found no residues in 1 sample of Turkish figs.

**Known 'nasty' pesticides used on or around figs:** CHLORPYRIFOS, CYPERMETHRIN, DDT, DELTAMETHRIN, DIELDRIN, GAMMA-HCH.

**Other possibly hazardous pesticides used:** ETHION, PHOSALONE, FENPROPIMORPH, MALATHION, PIRIMIPHOS-METHYL.

**Fish** In the UK in 1988 the average person consumed 3.9 lb of fresh fish; 1.7 lb of processed and shelled fish; 5.72 lb of prepared fish and fish products and over 5 lb of frozen fish. In the UK in 1988/9 a wide range of imported Chinese canned and dried fish was found to contain organochlorines including gamma-HCH, DDT and ppDDE. In 1990 laboratory tests revealed the presence of dichlorvos in salmon sold in UK shops.

Fish in California in 1985 were found to be contaminated with DDT dumped near a sewer discharge area. Although the levels of this organo-chlorine pesticide may be dropping in many parts of the world, similar problems to the Californian one may exist.

In 1988 in the US, 72% of domestic fish and shellfish sampled contained pesticide residues and 2% were over US tolerances.** For fish and shellfish imported into the US the figure was 23%.

In Australia, DDT was found in canned tuna, PCBs in imported tuna, and fenitrothion, chlorpyrifos-methyl and pirimiphos-methyl in fish.

The pesticides cited here are the most worrying ones of the many which have been found to contaminate fish. In the UK in 1984-5 very low levels of organo-chlorine pesticide residues were detected in fish in the typical UK person's diet.

**Known 'nasty' pesticides which may be used on or around the fish or with which they may come into contact:** DICHLORVOS, DDT, PCBS.

Other possibly hazardous pesticides which may be used on or around the fish or with which they may come into contact: Residues of many pesticides which enter fresh and salt water; also FENITROTHION, CHLORPYRIFOS-METHYL, PIRIMIPHOS-METHYL.

## Flageolet beans (see Beans)

## Forage crops (and Fodder crops which may be consumed indirectly by humans in the food chain. See also Corn, Peanuts, Beans) In the UK in 1987 it was found that of 10 samples of alfalfa seed, 8 contained inorganic bromides. In 1988, in 44 samples of cattle feed tested, 17 contained gamma-HCH, 3 ppDDE and 2 endosulfan. For pig feed the figures were 19 samples, 3 with gamma-HCH, 1 at MRL level**. For poultry feed, 31 samples were taken, 10 contained gamma-HCH, 1 over the MRL**, 1 contained dieldrin, 1 ppDDT and 1 op-DDT.

Known 'nasty' pesticides used on or around the crops: Large numbers of insecticides, herbicides, growth regulators and fungicides including CARBARYL, DIMETHOATE, METHYL PARATHION, PHOSMET.

Other possibly hazardous pesticides used: CARBOFURAN, CHLORPYRIFOS, DIAZINON, MALATHION, METHIDATHION, METHOXYCHLOR, PARATHION.

## Fowl (see also Poultry) In the UK in 1988/9, 1 sample of pheasant contained residues of dieldrin in excess of UK MRL** and one sample of woodpigeon was over the MRL for DDT** and dieldrin**. Of 15 pheasant samples, 4 contained gamma-HCH, 5 ppDDE, 1 dieldrin and 1 ppDDT.

There is some evidence in the UK to show that in the past chickens kept on wood shavings treated with wood preservatives like pentachlorophenol (see Part 3) will absorb the wood preservative into their liver and eggs.

In the US, it is acknowledged that meat, fish and poultry are second only to dairy products in their dietary contribution to the total adult intake of organo-chlorine pesticides.

Pesticide residues may occur in fowl because of the presence of pesticides or their metabolites on the foods eaten by fowl (vegetable or animal) or in buildings and materials in which fowl are kept.

## French beans (see Beans)

# Garlic

**Known 'nasty' pesticides used on or around garlic:** ALACHLOR (ASIA), CAPTAFOL (PACIFIC), CARBARYL (ASIA), CARBOSULFAN (ASIA), CHLOROTHALONIL, MANCOZEB (PACIFIC), MANEB (PACIFIC), METOLACHLOR (ASIA), TRIAZOPHOS (ASIA).

**Other possibly hazardous pesticides used:** AMITRAZ, ANILAZINE, CHLO-RFLUAZURON, DCNA, DIFLUBENZURON, IPRODIONE, MITC, OXADIAZON (ASIA), OXAMYL, PEN-DIMETHALIN (ASIA), PHOSALONE (ASIA), SULPHUR, TEFLUBENZURON.

**Goats** In the UK in 1988/9 of 31 samples of UK produced goats milk analysed, 6 samples contained pesticide residues: 4 of gamma-HCH, 1 of dieldrin, 1 of ppDDE. 21 different pesticides were sought.

**Known 'nasty' pesticides which may be used on or around goats:** These could include a whole range of insecticides, herbicides, growth regulators and fungicides.

# Gooseberries

**Known 'nasty' pesticides used on or around gooseberries:** AZINPHOS-METHYL, BENOMYL, CARBARYL, CARBENDAZIM, CHLOROTHALONIL, CHLORPYRIFOS, CYPER-METHRIN, DINOCAP, DSM, MANCOZEB, O-DM, PARAQUAT, NICOTINE.

**Other possibly hazardous pesticides used:** BORDEAUX MIXTURE, BUPIRIMATE, CHLORPROPHAM, CHLORTHAL-DIMETHYL, COPPER HYDROXIDE, COPPER SULPHATE, CUFRANEB, CYFLUTHRIN, DALAPON, 2,4-DES, DICHLOBENIL, DICHLOFLUANID, DIMETHOATE, DIURON, DODINE, FENAMINOL, FENITROTHION, FLUAZIFOP-METHYL, HEPTENOPHOS, ISOX-ABEN, LENACIL, MALATHION, NAPROPAMIDE, OXADIAZON, PENDIMETHALIN, PENTANCHLOR, PIRIMICARB, PROPYZAMIDE, PYRETHRINS, ROTENONE, SULPHUR, SIMAZINE, SODIUM MONO-CHLOROACETATE, SULPHUR, TAR OILS, TETRADIFON, TRIADIMEFOM, TRIFORINE, VINCLOZOLIN.

**Grapefruit** In the UK in 1988/9 13 out of 25 imported grapefruit samples contained multi-residues and 22 pesticides were sought: 9 contained biphenyl, 15 thiabendazole, 1 chlor-pyrifos, 3 2,4-D, 2 ethion and 3 methidathion, but none exceeded MRLs. Residues detected came from Cyprus, Israel, Spain, the US and South Africa.

Some Israeli growers now supply UK shops with organic grapefruit.

In Canada in 1986/7 low levels of benomyl were detected in imported fruit. In Sweden in 1989 14 out of 54 samples of imported fruit contained residues including biphenyl, carbaryl, chlorpyrifos, ethion, imazalil, methidathion, metalaxyl and thiabendazole.

In the US, the NRDC found that of the residues detected in grapefruit, thiabendazole, ethion, carbaryl and chlorobenzilate residues could all be reduced by washing, but the effects of washing on methidathion were unknown.

**Known 'nasty' pesticides used on or around grapefruit:** AZINPHOS-METHYL, BROMACIL, CARBARYL, CHLOROBENZILATE, CHLORPYRIFOS, CYHEXATIN, DICOFOL, DIMETHO-ATE, DIURON, METHOMYL, PARAQUAT, PARATHION.

**Other possibly hazardous pesticides used:** 2,4-D, ETHION, GLYPHOSATE, IMAZALIL, MALATHION, METALAXYL, METHIOCARB, METHIDATHION, THIABENDAZOLE.

**Grapes** *(including Currants, Raisins and Sultanas. See also* **Wine***)*
In 1989, the average Briton consumed over $2^{1}/_{2}$ lb of fresh grapes.

In a UK sample of 36 imported currant shipments, 2 contained diazinon, 2 carbendazim, 1 ppDDT, 1 ppDDE and 5 inorganic bromide: Greek currants contained most residues followed by South Africa. For raisins, in a sample of 47, 2 contained gamma-HCH, 3 ppDDT, 3 opDDT, 1 ppDDE, 1 permethrin, 16 inorganic bromide: most residues were detected in American, Afghanistan and South African raisins. For sultanas, in a sample of 42, 5 contained gamma-HCH, 3 ppDDT, 1 carbendazim, 13 inorganic bromide: most were from Greece and Australia.

In Australia in 1987 DDT and dicofol were found in sultanas.

In 1985 California found demetron-methyl in the wines from one producer. There was a demeton-methyl tolerance level for grapes but not wine. Although the levels found were evaluated as not harmful, this again reveals gaps in our knowledge and control of pesticide residues in a range of foods.

In 1988 the US detained grapes from one Italian shipper because of one pesticide residue. In the same year, of those grapes imported into the US and sampled, 48% contained pesticide residues but none over US tolerance levels. In 1986 the Danes found grapes from Spain exceeded Danish MRLs on mono-crotophos**. The US NRDC found that of the residues found in grapes in that country, captan, dicloran and carbaryl residues could be reduced by washing but the effects of washing on iprodione and dimethoate residues are unknown.

In Sweden in 1989, of 140 samples of imported grapes, 42 contained residues including captan/folpet, acephate, carbaryl, carbendazim, cypermethrin, diazinon, EBDCs, parathion, meth-amidophos, omethoate and monocrotophos. Greek grapes exceeded Swedish MRLs on monocrotophos**, Italian grapes exceeded Swedish MRLs on EBDCs**, carbendazim** and omethoate**; Turkish grapes exceeded Swedish MRLs on monocrotophos** and carbendazim**.

In 1988, of domestic US grapes sampled, 28% contained pesticide residues but none over US tolerance levels.

In 1988/89 Canada recorded a single shipment of US grapes containing excessive levels of vinclozolin (*Food Chemicals News*, 21 May, 1990). In Canada in 1986/7 benomyl was detected at low levels in imported grapes as were azinphos-methyl, captan, folpet, iprodione, parathion, phosalone, phosmet and tetradifon. In the same years, Canada detected imported grapes above Canadian MRLs: 1% broke MRLs on acephate**, 5% on chlorpyrifos**, 4% on dimethoate**.

In India in 1989 it was reported that DDT and BHC had been detected in grapes in past surveys.

**Known 'nasty' pesticides used on or around grapes:** CARBENDAZIM, CAPTAN, CHLOROTHALONIL, CHLORPYRIFOS, CYPERMETHRIN, DELTAMETHRIN, DIELDRIN, DINOCAP (SOUTH AFRICA), ENDOSULFAN (SOUTH AFRICA), FOLPET (SOUTH AFRICA), GAMMA-HCH, HCB, MANCOZEB, METIRAM (SOUTH AFRICA), PARAQUAT.

**Other possibly hazardous pesticides used:** BORDEAUX MIXTURE, COPPER OXYCHLORIDE, COPPER SULPHATE, CUFRAMEB, DICHLOFLUANID, DIMETHOATE, DIQUAT, ETHION, FENARIMOL, FENTHION (SOUTH AFRICA), FENVALERATE, GLYPHOSATE, IPRODIONE, MALATHION, METALAXYL, METHIOCARB, OXADIAZON, PERMETHRIN, PETROLEUM OIL, PHOSALONE, PROCYMIDONE, PROPOXUR (SOUTH AFRICA), PROPYZAMIDE, SIMAZINE, SULPHUR, TRIADIMEFON, VINCLOZOLIN.

Grape pests can be controlled by integrated pest management techniques which do not require the use of pesticides. For instance, the grape leafhopper in California has been controlled by leafhopper egg parasites. These effective parasites survive the winter months because growers encourage blackberry hoppers on which the parasites can feed.

**Guavas** In India in 1989 it was reported that DDT and BHC had been detected in the fruit in the past.

**Known 'nasty' pesticides used on or around guavas:** ALDICARB (SOUTH AFRICA), CHLORDANE (SOUTH AFRICA), CHLORPYRIFOS (SOUTH AFRICA), CYPERMETHRIN (SOUTH AFRICA), DELTAMETHRIN (SOUTH AFRICA), DIAZINON (PACIFIC), DICHLORVOS (SOUTH AFRICA), PARATHION (SOUTH AFRICA), MANCOZEB (SOUTH AFRICA), METHOMYL (SOUTH AFRICA), MEVINPHOS (SOUTH AFRICA), OMETHOATE (SOUTH AFRICA).

**Other possibly hazardous pesticides used:** FENTHION (SOUTH AFRICA), MAL-ATHION (PACIFIC), TRIADIMEFON, TRICHLORFON (SOUTH AFRICA), TRIFORINE (SOUTH AFRICA).

## Ham *(see Pork)*

## Herbs In the UK in 1986 82% of a representative sample of herbs was found to have been treated with herbicides.

In 1986 in Denmark, EBDCs** were found on chives above the Danish MRL levels.

**Known 'nasty' pesticides used on or around herbs:** DELTAMETHRIN, DSM.

**Other possibly hazardous pesticides used:** CHLORTHAL-DIMETHYL, CLOPYRALID, DIQUAT, LENACIL, LINURON, PROPACHLOR, PROPYZAMIDE, TRIFLURALIN.

## Honey In 1989 the average Briton ate ³/₄ lb of honey.

In 1988/9, of 7 samples of UK honey checked by MAFF, gamma-HCH was present in 1 sample and 17 residues were sought. No residues were found in 1 sample of imported honey.

In Bombay, honey was found to contain BHC, gamma-HCH, heptachlor and aldrin/dieldrin but not above the WHO tolerances.

**Pesticides which may be found in honey:** CYPERMETHRIN, DDT, DELTAMETHRIN, DIELDRIN, FENVALERATE, FENPROPATHRIN, GAMMA-HCH, HEPTACHLOR, MALATHION, PIRIMIPHOS-METHYL.

## Hops *(see also Beer)* 95% of UK hops would not be acceptable in the US because of the wide and extensive use of pesticides on hops (see Parratt and Patton). Since 1986, Czechoslovakia has rejected some beers produced domestically because of pyrethroid residues. In Germany, beers are checked for 33 different residues but even up to 1989 this was not common practice in the UK. Some organic hops from Germany and Tasmania are exported.

**Known 'nasty' pesticides used on or around hops:** ALDICARB, BENOMYL, CHLOROTHALONIL, CARBENDAZIM, CYPERMETHRIN, DICOFOL, DIMETHOATE, DELTAMETHRIN, DINOCAP, DSM, ENDOSULFAN, GAMMA-HCH, NICOTINE, PARAQUAT, ZINEB.

**Other possibly hazardous pesticides used:** AMITRAZ, ASULAM, BORDEAUX MIX-TURE, BUPIRIMATE, COPPER HYDROXIDE, COPPER OXYCHLORIDE, COPPER SULPHATE, DI-QUAT, FOSETYL-ALUMINIUM, FENVALERATE, MEPHOSFOLAN, METALAXYL, OXADIAZON, OMETHOATE, PENDIMETHALIN, PENCONAZOLE, PROPYZAMIDE, PYRAZOPHOS, SIMAZINE, SO-DIUM MONOCHLOROACETATE, SULPHUR, TAR OILS, TETRADIFON, TRIADIMEFON, TRIFORINE.

**Horse radish** In 1986 in the UK, 57% of a representative sample of horse radish had been treated with insecticides, 100% with fungicides and 100% with herbicides.

## Ice cream (see Beef and dairy products)

**Kale** In 1986 in the UK, in a representative sample of kale and broccoli, 88% had been treated with insecticides, 53% with seed treaments, 43% with fungicides and 94% with herbicides.

In 1988 the US detained kale from one Mexican shipper for one pesticide residue. In the same year 85% of a sample of 41 imported kale plants contained pesticide residues.

**Known 'nasty' pesticides used on or around kale:** ALDICARB, BENOMYL, CARBEN-DAZIM, CARBOFURAN, CYPERMETHRIN, DELTAMETHRIN, DINOCAP, DIMETHOATE, FONOFOS, GAMMA-HCH, MANEB, THIRAM, ZINEB.

**Other possibly hazardous pesticides used:** ALLOXYDIM-SODIUM, CARBOSULFAN, CHLORFENVINPHOS, CLOPYRALID, COPPER SULPHATE, DALAPON, DI-1-P-METHANE, FLUAZIFOP-P-BUTYL, METAZACHLOR, PIRIMICARB, POTASSIUM SORBATE, PROPACHLOR, PYRAZOPHOS, SETHOXYDIM, SODIUM METABISULPHITE, SODIUM PROPIONATE, SULPHUR, TCA, TEBUTAM, THIABENDAZOLE, TRIADIMEFON, TRICHLORFON.

**Kiwi fruit** Sweden in 1989 looked at 42 samples of kiwi fruit and found 9 contained pesticides. 2 contained organophosphorous pesticides, 1 captan/folpet, 1 chlorothanil over the Swedish MRL** , 3 chlorpyrifos, 1 diazinon, 1 dicofol, 1 iprodione, 2 methidathion, 1 pirimiphos-methyl and 4 vinclozolin. It was Italian fruit that exceeded the Swedish MRL.

## Kohl rabi

**Known 'nasty' pesticides used on or around kohl rabi:** MANEB, ZINEB.

**Other possibly hazardous pesticide used:** SULPHUR.

**Kumquat** In the UK in 1988/9 a sample of 10 imported kumquats was tested for 22 different pesticides and 1 of these, from the US, contained 2-aminobutane. No residues were detected in Israeli or other US fruit.

## Lamb (see Sheep)

**Leeks** In the UK in 1988, in a representative sample of leeks, 26% of the crop had been treated with insecticides, 35% with pesticidal seed treatments, 61% with fungicides and 85% with herbicides.

In 1988, 7% of a US sample of 15 imported leeks contained pesticide residues.

In Sweden in 1989, 25 imported leek samples were tested for residues; 2 from Holland contained chlorothalonil over Swedish MRLs**, 1 contained EBDCs and 1 parathion.

**Known 'nasty' pesticides used on or around leeks:** ALDICARB, BENOMYL, CAPTAN, CARBENDAZIM, CHLOROTHALONIL, CYPERMETHRIN, DELTAMETHRIN, DIMETHOATE, DSM, FOLPET, IOXYNIL, MALEIC HYDRAZIDE, MANCOZEB, MANEB, MERCUROUS CHLORIDE, NICOTINE, TRIALLATE, ZINEB.

**Other possibly hazardous pesticides used:** ALLOXYDIM-SODIUM, AZIPROTRYNE, BENTAZONE, BROMPHOS, CARBOFURAN, CHLORBUFAM, CHLORPROPHAM, CHLORIDAZON, CHLORTHAL-DIMETHYL, CLOPYRALID, COPPER HYDROXIDE, CYANAZINE, DICLOFOP-METHYL, FENITROTHION, FENPROPIMORPH, FENURON, FERBAM, HEPTENOPHOS, IODEFENPHOS, IPRO-DIONE, MALATHION, METALAXYL, METHAM-SODIUM, MONOLINURON, OXAMYL, PEN-DIMETHALIN, PROMETRYN, PROPACHLOR, PROPAMOCARB HYDROCHLORIDE, PYRETHRINS, SETHOXYDIM, SODIUM MONOCHLOROACETATE, THIABENDAZOLE, THIRAM, TRIADIMEFON, TRI-AZOPHOS, VINCLOZOLIN.

**Lemons** *(see also Waxes)* In the UK in 1986/7, 15 samples of cut mixed peel were tested for residues, 3 (2 from Italy and 1 from Netherlands) contained 2-phenylphenol and 1 from Italy contained thiabendazole. In 1988/9 multiple residues were found in 4 samples of lemon and of 13 samples tested for 22 pesticides the UK found 3 with biphenyl, 1 with fenitrothion, 11 with parathion-methyl, 3 with 2, phenylphenol and 2 with thiabendazole. Residues were detected in imports from Cyprus, Spain and the US, but none was detected in the 1 Turkish sample analysed.

In Sweden in 1989, 44 imported samples of lemon were examined; 16 had residues. These were azinphos-methyl, biphenyl, carbendazim, chlorfenvinphos, dicofol, endosulfan, ethion, mecarbam, methidathion and metalaxyl.

In 1987 low levels of benomyl were detected in lemons imported into Canada.

In 1988 the US detained lemons from 5 Spanish shippers because of two pesticide residues.

In 1987 Denmark found that lemons from Spain exceeded Danish MRLs**.

**Known 'nasty' pesticides used on or around lemons:** AZINPHOS-METHYL, BENOMYL, CARBENDAZIM, CARBOSULFAN, DICOFOL, ENDOSULFAN, PARATHION-METHYL.

**Other possibly hazardous pesticides used:** BIPHENYLS, CHLORFENVINPHOS, CYFLUTHRIN, ETHION, FENITROTHION, FENVALERATE, MECARBAM, METALAXYL, METH-IDATHION, THIABENDAZOLE.

The effect of alcohol on pesticide residues in fruit is not clearly understood. Some commentators suggest that alcohol could increase the toxic effects of pesticide residues on lemon slices in drinks. Others suggest that the toxic effects of the alcohol are a greater cause for concern than any residues. We can perhaps look forward to a time when supermarkets label accurately both the contents of a bottle of gin, a bottle of bitter lemon and a fresh lemon and indicate possible hazards presented by consuming all three simultaneously.

**Lentils** In 1986 and 1987, samples of pulses were taken from UK retail outlets. 10 out of 25 lentil samples were found to contain pesticide residues. Pesticides detected in the 10 samples included gamma-HCH, DDT metabolites, tecnazene, malathion and pirimiphos-methyl.

**Pesticides which may be used on or around the crop:** these are numerous and include METALAXYL.

**Lettuce** The average Briton eats over 6 lb of fresh leafy salad a year. The average American eats 11 lb of lettuce a year.

In the UK in 1986, of a representative sample of lettuce crops, it was found that 88% had been treated with insecticide, 24% with molluscicides, 42% with fungicides, 87% with herbicides. In 1988/9, 77 UK lettuce samples and 24 imported lettuce samples were tested for 21 different residues. Multiple residues were found in 42 samples. UK lettuces contained 2 samples above the CAC MRL**, 16 imported samples contained EBDCs in excess of the proposed CAC MRL**, 3 samples of lettuce contained DSM residues above the proposed CAC MRL**, 14 UK lettuces exceeded the CAC MRL in inorganic bromide**. 4 samples of UK lettuce contained residues of more than 1 pesticide above a confirmed or proposed MRL**. In the 77 domestic samples tested, 75 contained metalaxyl, 77 inorganic bromide, 36 EBDCs, 29 tolclofos-methyl, 26 iprodione, 6 DSM, 5 dimethoate and 4 cypermethrin.

In 1988 the US detained one Belgium shipper's leaf lettuce because of pesticide residues. In the same year in the US 50% of a sample of 153 imported lettuces contained pesticide residues and 1% of the sample exceeded US tolerance levels.

Canada in 1986 found 1% of its domestic lettuces tested exceeded the MRL for permethrin**. In 1988/9 they expressed concern about lettuce from the US and Mexico and monitored levels of acephate, ethion, chlordimeform, peremethrin and methamidophos closely. In 1987 Spanish lettuces exceeded Danish MRLs on certain pesticides**.

In 1989 in Sweden, of 16 imported lettuce samples checked, 6 contained residues and some Dutch lettuces exceeded Swedish MRLs on inorganic bromide**. Domestic Swedish lettuces exceeded Swedish MRLs on malathion, mevinphos and acephate**.

In Poland between 1986-88, residues of EBDCs** were detected in lettuces above Polish MRLs; also detected were MBC and iprodione.

If outer leaves are discarded this may reduce the presence of some pesticide on lettuce. The US NRDC found washing also reduced permethrin levels found on the salad but did not reduce methomyl and mevinphos.

**Known 'nasty' pesticides used on or around lettuce:** BENOMYL, CAPTAN, CARBARYL, CARBENDAZIM, CYPERMETHRIN, DICHLORVOS, DIMETHOATE, DISULFOTON, DSM, GAMMA-HCH, MANCOZEB, METHOMYL, NALED, NICOTINE, OXYDEMETON METHYL, PARATHION, PHORATE, THIRAM, ZINEB.

**Other possibly hazardous pesticides used:** CETRIMIDE, CHLORPROPHAM, DCNA, DIAZINON, DICLOFOP-METHYL, DICLORAN, DIURON, FERBAM, FOSETYL-ALUMINIUM, HEPTENPHOS, IPRODIONE, MALATHION, METALAXYL, METHOXYCHLOR, MEVINPHOS, PERMETHRIN, PIRIMICARB, PROPACHLOR, PROPHAM, PROPYRAMIDE, PYRETHRINS, QUINTOZENE, RESMETHRIN, SULPHUR, TECNAZENE, TOLCLOFOS-METHYL, TRICHLORFON, TRIFLURALIN, VINCLOZOLIN.

## Lima beans (see Beans)

## Maize (See Corn)

## Mangetout

**Known 'nasty' pesticides used on or around mangetout:** DSM, NICOTINE, THIRAM.

**Other possibly hazardous pesticides used:** DRAZOXOLON, IPRODIONE, MCPB, METALAXYL, THIABENDAZOLE, TRIALLATE.

**Mangoes** In Sweden in 1989, of 19 imported samples of mango, 4 contained carbendazim, EBDCs, omethoate and thiabendazole residues.

In India in 1989 residues of DDT and BHC were reported in mangoes.

**Known 'nasty' pesticides used on or around mangoes:** BENOMYL, CAPTAN, CARBARYL, CYHEXATIN, CYPERMETHRIN, DIAZINON, DELTAMETHRIN, DICOFOL, MANCOZEB, MANEB, MONOCROTOPHOS, PARATHION, ZINEB.

**Other possibly hazardous pesticides used:** CYFLUTHRIN, DIFLUBENZURON, FENTHION, FENVALERATE, MALATHION, PERMETHRIN, TRIDEMORPH.

**Marrows** In 1986, of a representative sample of UK marrows, 14% had been treated with insecticides, 77% with seed treatments, 82% with fungicides, 59% with herbicides and only 11% had been treated with nothing.

**Known 'nasty' pesticides used on or around marrows:** CYPERMETHRIN, DIMETHOATE, DSM, DISULFOTON, MANEB, NICOTINE, TRIAZOPHOS, ZINEB.

**Other possibly hazardous pesticides used:** BENDIOCARB, BUPIRIMATE, DIPHENAMID, HEPTENOPHOS, IMAZALIL, IPRODIONE, OXAMYL, PIRIMICARB, PROPAMOCARB HYDROCHLORIDE, PYRAZOPHOS, THIABENDAZOLE, THIRAM.

**Melons** *(see also **Water melons**)* In 1988 the US detained bitter melons from seven Dominican shippers because of one pesticide residue, and honeydew melons from one Panama shipper because of one pesticide residue. Of 105 bitter melons imported into the US in 1988 and sampled, 22% contained pesticide residues but none over US tolerance levels. Of 104 imported honeydew melons sampled, 62% contained pesticide residues.

In 1988 in the US 42% of domestic honeydew melons sampled contained pesticide residues but none over tolerance levels.

In 1988 in the US 27% of domestic cantaloupes sampled contained pesticide residues but none exceeded the US tolerance. Of fruit imported into the US, 62% contained pesticide residues from a sample of 338. In 1988 the US detained cantaloupes from one Costa Rican, one Honduran and one Guatemalan shipper each because of pesticide residues.

The NRDC have detected a number of residues on cantaloupes of which only chlorothalonil can be washed off; methamidophos cannot, and the effects of washing on endosulfan, dimethoate and methyl parathion are unknown.

In 1987/8 a small percentage of melons imported into Canada contained residues of methomyl, dimethoate, endosulfan and methamidophos.

In Sweden in 1989, of 40 imported melon samples tested, 4 contained residues of captan/folpet, acephate, endosulfan, methamidophos and monocrotophos.

**Known 'nasty' pesticides used on or around melons:** AZINPHOS-METHYL, BENOMYL, CAPTAN, CARBARYL, CARBOFURAN, CARBOSULFAN, CHLOROTHALONIL, DIAZINON, DICOFOL, DIMETHOATE, DINOCAP, ENDOSULFAN, MANCOZEB, MANEB, METHOMYL, MEVINPHOS, NALED, ODM.

**Ohter possibly hazardous pesticides used:** BENFURACARB, CHLORTHAL-DIMETHYL, COPPER, ETHION, ESFENVALERATE, FENVALERATE, MALATHION, METALAXYL, METHIOCARB, METHOMYL, METHOXYCHLOR, PHOSPHAMIDON, TETRADIFON, TRIADIMEFON, TRIDEMORPH, TRICHLORFON.

**Milk** *(see also **Beef and dairy produce**)* In 1989, each person in the UK consumed on average over 123 pints of fresh milk and cream and over 56 pints of skimmed milk.

In 1988 in the UK residues of organochlorines were detected in 44% of 120 samples of milk. The figure for 1989 was 12% in a sample of 126. All levels were below the UK MRLs. In 1988 sampled milk sold in the UK contained residues of HCB, HCH isomers, dieldrin and ppDDE. Other residues were recorded but not above their reporting levels – these included chlordane, iodofenphos, phosmet, dichlorvos, diazinon and endrin.

In 1989 sampled milk sold in the UK contained residues of HCH isomers, dieldrin and ppDDE. Other residues were recorded but not above reporting levels – these included, in addition to several listed for 1988, permethrin, deltamethrin, cypermethrin, atrazine, simazine and cyanzine.

In the 1980s, the US accepted that dairy products were the main dietary source of organo-chlorine residues in the total adult intake of those chemicals.

**Mung beans** *(see Beans)*

**Mushrooms** The average Briton eats over 3 lb of fresh mushrooms a year. In 1986 Denmark found carbendazim levels in their domestic mushrooms above Danish MRLs**. In Sweden in 1989 1 sample of 11 imported mushroom batches contained imazalil residues. In Poland between 1986 and 1988 residues of MBC were found in mushrooms.

In 1983 and 1984, 15 of 120 mushroom samples taken direct from UK growers contained pesticide residues of which 2 exceeded CAC or EC MRLs for DDT**.

The US in 1988 detained mushrooms from one shipper in France and one shipper in the Netherlands because of one pesticide residue each.

**Known 'nasty' pesticides used on or around mushrooms:** BENOMYL, CARBENDAZIM, CHLOROTHALONIL, DELTAMETHRIN, DIAZINON, DICHLORVOS, METHYL BROMIDE, METHOXYCHLOR, NICOTINE, ZINEB.

**Other possibly hazardous pesticides used:** CHLORFENVINPHOS, DICHLOROPHEN, DIFLUBENZURON, MALATHION, PERMETHRIN, PIRIMIPHOS-ETHYL, PIRIMIPHOS-METHYL, PROCHLORAZ, RESMETHRIN, SODIUM PENTACHLOROPHENOXIDE, THIABENDAZOLE.

**Mustard** Mustard may be used as a fodder crop or for direct human consumption.

In 1988 in the US 79% of a sample of 14 imported mustard greens contained pesticide residues and 7% of the sample exceeded US tolerance levels**.

**Known 'nasty' pesticides used on or around mustard:** CARBARYL, DIMETHOATE, DSM, ENDOSULFAN, MANEB, PARATHION.

**Other possibly hazardous pesticides used:** MALATHION, METHOMYL, MEVINPHOS. ON UK MUSTARD: AZINPHOS-METHYL, BENAZOLIN, CLOPYRALID, DICLOFOP-METHYL, DIQUAT, GLYPHOSATE, IPRODIONE, MALATHION, PHOSALONE, PROPYZAMIDE, TCA, TRIALLATE, TRIAZOPHOS, TRIFLURALIN.

## Mutton (see Sheep)

**Nectarines** In Canada in 1988/9 a sample of 19 imported nectarine batches was analysed and residues of dimethyl formamide were found in 8 and triforine in 12.

In Sweden in 1989 Italian nectarines exceeded Swedish MRLs on acephate and methamidophos**. 13 of 40 imports also contained chlorpyrifos, dicloran, EBDCs and pirimicarb.

In 1988 in the US 49% of 49 domestic nectarines sampled contained pesticide residues but none exceeded US tolerance levels. The figure for imported fruit was 96% with none over tolerance levels.

**Known 'nasty' pesticides used on or around nectarines:** AMINOTRIAZOLE, DSM, ODM.

**Other possibly hazardous pesticides used:** ASULAM, BORDEAUX MIXTURE, COPPER HYDROXIDE, COPPER OXYCHLORIDE, COPPER SULPHATE, CUFRANEB, CUPRIC AMMONIUM CARBONATE, TAR OILS, TETRADIFON, VINCLOZOLIN.

**Nuts** *(see also Peanuts)* In 1989 the average person in the UK consumed over 1½ lb of nuts and nut produce.

In the UK in 1988/9, 160 samples of nuts were analysed for residues. The table shows the results:

| Nuts | Number analysed | Residues found | No. of samples affected |
|---|---|---|---|
| almonds | 28 | malathion (1), methacrifos (1), pirimiphos-methyl (1), inorganic bromide | 24 |
| brazil | 22 | gamma-HCH (1), inorganic bromide | 22 |
| cashew | 21 | gamma-HCH (3), malathion (1), inorganic bromide | 5 |
| chestnuts | 8 | inorganic bromide | 3 |
| hazel | 17 | ppDDE (1) | 5 |
| peanuts | 22 | HCH isomers including gamma-HCH (9), malathion (1), inorganic bromide | 18 |
| pine | 5 | gamma-HCH (1), malathion (1), inorganic bromide | 1 |
| pistachio | 4 | | 4 |
| tiger | 4 | ppDDE (1) | 4 |
| walnuts | 24 | gamma-HCH (1) | 21 |

In 1988 in the US, 23% of imported cashew nuts, from 14 samples, contained pesticide residues.

**Known 'nasty' pesticides used on or around nuts:** ALDICARB, AZINPHOS-METHYL, BENOMYL, CAPTAN, CARBARYL, CARBOPHENOTHION, CHLOROPICRIN, CHLORPYRIFOS-METHYL, CYPERMETHRIN, DDT, DIURON, ETHION, ENDOSULFAN, GAMMA-HCH, HEPTACHLOR, METHYL BROMIDE, PARATHION, PARAQUAT, PHOSMET.

**Other possibly hazardous pesticides used:** ATRAZINE, DODINE, ESFENVALERATE, FENVALERATE, GLYPHOSATE, MALATHION, METHACRIFOS, PIRIMIPHOS-METHYL, PROPICONAZOLE, THIOPHANATE-METHYL.

Nut pests can be controlled by non-chemical means. For instance, the walnut aphid in Californa has been successfully controlled by a parasitic wasp introduced from Iran.

**Oats** The average Briton eats 2 lb of oats a year.

In 1985-6, 71 samples of processed oats were analysed in the UK for residues. 13 contained residues, including chlorpyrifos-methyl, pirimiphos-methyl and malathion.

**Known 'nasty' pesticides used on or around oats:** AMITROLE, BENOMYL, BROMOXYNIL, CARBENDAZIM, CHLOROTHALONIL, CHLORPYRIFOS, CYPERMETHRIN, DELTAMETHRIN, DSM, EBDCS, FONOFOS, GAMMA-HCH, IOXYNIL, MANCOZEB, MANEB, OMETHOATE, OXYDEMETON-METHYL, PARAQUAT, TRIAZOPHOS, ZINEB.

**Other possibly hazardous pesticides used:** BENODANIL, CHLORMEQUAT, CLOPYRALID, CYNAZINE, 2,4-D, DALAPON, DICAMBA, DICHLOBENIL, ETHIRIMOL, FENITHROTHION, FENPROPIMORPH, FERBAM, FLUTRIAFOL, GLYPHOSATE, IMAZALIL, IPRODIONE, ISOPROTURON, LINURON, MALATHION, MCPA, MECOPROP, METOXURON, PENDIMETHALIN, PIRIMIPHOS-METHYL, PROPICONAZOLE, PROCHLORAZ, SIMAZINE, SULPHUR, TCA, TERBUTRYN, THIABENDAZOLE, THIOPHANATE-METHYL, THIRAM, TRIADIMENOL, TRIDEMORPH, TRIFORINE.

**Oils, vegetable** In the UK in 1988 the average person consumed 4.6 lb of vegetable and salad oils.

In 1988 in the US, 22% of a sample of 75 crude vegetable oils contained pesticide residues; 35% of a sample of 170 imported refined oils contained pesticide residues and 9% of other vegetable oil products from a sample of 11 imported contained pesticide residues.

**Okra** In 1988 the US detained okra from eight Dominican shippers because of four different pesticide residues. Of 159 okra plants imported and sampled in the US in 1988, 26% contained pesticide residues.

**Known 'nasty' pesticides which may be used on or around okra:** CARBARYL, CARBOFURAN, ETHYLENE DIBROMIDE, METHYL BROMIDE, MEVINPHOS, PARATHION.

**Other possibly hazardous pesticides used:** MALATHION, METALAXYL, MITC.

**Olives**

**Known 'nasty' pesticides used on or around olives:** AZINPHOS-METHYL, DSM, MANCOZEB.

Chemicals are not necessary to control some pests of the olive. Olive scale has been controlled in California by the use of its natural enemies introduced from India, Pakistan and Iran.

**Onions** The average Briton consumes over $11^1/_2$ lb of fresh onions, shallots and leeks each year.

Over 46 different countries export onions.

In 1986 in the UK, of a representative sample of onions, 52% of dry onions had been treated with insecticide, 79% received seed treatment, 79% fungicides, 99% herbicides and 52% growth regulators. The figures for salad onions were 26% treated with insecticides, 88% with seed treatments, 59% with fungicides and 81% with herbicides.

In the UK in 1988/9, samples of 24 bulb onions and 22 imported onions were tested for 8 different pesticides: maleic hydrazide was detected in 10 domestic samples and in 3 imported samples (all from Spain).

In Poland between 1986-88 residues of EBDCs and diazinon were detected above Polish MRLs**. In Canada in 1988/9, a small number of 89 domestic onion samples contained residues of sethoxydim and its metabolites. In Sweden in 1989, no residues were detected in 47 samples of imported onions.

In 1988 in the US, 21% of a sample of 85 imported onions contained pesticide residues. For the same year 10% of a sample of 20 imported shallots contained pesticide residues. The EPA registered 50 pesticides for use on onions and the FDA can routinely identify 60% of those. The NRDC found residues of DCPA, DDT, ethion, diazinon and malathion on onions: of these DDT, ethion and malathion could be reduced by washing.

**Known 'nasty' pesticides used on or around onions:** ALACHLOR, ALDICARB, BENOMYL, CAPTAN, CARBENDAZIM, CARBOFURAN, CHLOROTHALONIL, CYPERMETHRIN, DELTAMETHRIN, DIMETHOATE, DSM, IOXYNIL, MALEIC HYDRAZIDE, MANEB, METHYL PARATHION, NICOTINE, TRIALLATE, ZINEB.

**Other possibly hazardous pesticides used:** ALLOXYDIM-SODIUM, ANILAZINE, AZIPROTYRNE, BENTAZONE, BROMOPHOS, CHLORBUFAM, CHLORIDAZON, CHLORPROPHAM, CHLORTHAL-DIMETHYL, CLOPYRALID, COPPER HYDROXIDE, CYANAZINE, DCNA, DIAZINON, DICLOFOP-METHYL, FENITROTHION, FENPROPIMORPH, FENURON, FERBAM, FLUAZIFOP-P-BUTYL, HEPTENOPHOS, IODOFENPHOS, IPRODIONE, MALATHION, MERCUROUS CHLORIDE, METALAXYL, METHAM-SODIUM, MONOLINUON, OXADIAZON, OXAMYL, PENDIMETHALIN, PROMETRYN, PROPACHLOR, PROPAMCARB, PYRETHRINS, SETHOXYDIM, SODIUM MONOCHLOROACETATE, SULPHUR, THIABENDAZOLE, TRIADIMEFOM, TRIAZOPHOS, VINCLOZOLIN.

**Oranges** In 1989, each Briton consumed on average nearly 10 lb of fresh oranges. Average US consumption is 7 lb a year.

3% of oranges imported from the US into Canada in 1988/9 were in violation of Canada's pesticide residue standards**. The residues detected included carbofuran, chlorpyrifos, endosulfan and malathion on the skins. In 1986/7 low levels of benomyl were detected on oranges imported into Canada.

In 1986 Denmark found imported oranges exceeded Danish MRLs on azinphos-methyl** and parathion-methyl**.

In Sweden in 1989 some Spanish mandarin oranges exceeded Swedish MRLs on azinphos-methyl**, ones from the US did so on carbendazim**, some from Israel did so on ethion** and some from Morocco did so on fenthion** and parathion methyl**. Imported Moroccan oranges also contained residues of pirimicarb, parathion, metalaxyl, imazalil, diazinon, fenitrothion, methidathion and thiabendazole.

In 1988 in the US 63% of the domestic oranges sampled contained pesticide residues but none over US tolerance levels. The figure for oranges imported into the US was 46%. The EPA registers 90 pesticides for use on oranges and the FDA can routinely identify only 50% of those in residue tests.

Peeling oranges will remove some pesticide residues like carbaryl, ethion and parathion located in the peel.

**Known 'nasty' pesticides used on or around oranges:** AZINPHOS-METHYL, BENOMYL, BROMACIL, CAPTAFOL, CARBARYL, CARBENDAZIM, CARBOFURAN, CHLOROBENZILATE, CHLORPYRIFOS, DIAZINON, DICOFOL, DIMETHOATE, DINOSEB, DIOXATHION, ENDOSULFAN, METHOMYL, NALED, PARAQUAT, PARATHION.

**Other possibly hazardous pesticides used:** ETHION, FENITROTHION, FORMETANATE, FENBUTATIN OXIDE, FENTHION, IMAZALIL, MALATHION, METALAXYL, METHIDATHION, METHIOCARB, PIRIMICARB, SULPHUR, THIABENDAZOLE.

Pests of citrus fruits can be controlled by a number of methods which do not require chemicals. Citrus black fly has been controlled in Mexico by using a parasite, and biological controls have been successfully used against purple scale in the US, Mexico, Greece, Brazil, Peru and Cyprus.

**Papayas** In 1989 in Sweden some Costa Rican papayas exceeded the Swedish MRLs on imazalil**, and of 12 samples tested 4 contained pesticide residues which included thiabendazole.

**Known 'nasty' pesticides used on or around papayas:** CHLOROBENZILATE, DICOFOL, DIURON, MANCOZEB.

**Other possibly hazardous pesticides used:** AZOCYCLOTIN, COPPER OXYCHLORIDE, FENAMIPHOS, HYDROXY PHENYLBUTAN-3-ONE, MALATHION.

**Parsley** In the UK in 1986, 87% of a representative sample of parsley had been treated with an insecticide, 7% with a seed treatment, 14% with fungicides and 100% with herbicides.

In Sweden in 1989, no residues were found in 3 imported samples of parsley tested.

In 1988 in the US, 84% of a sample of 37 imported parsley plants contained pesticide residues and in 1989 imported parsley was found to contain heptachlor/chlordane.

**Known 'nasty' pesticides used on or around parsley:** ALDICARB, BENOMYL, CAPTAN, CARBOSULFAN, CHLORDANE, DISULFOTON, DSM, DIMETHOATE, HEPTACHLOR, MANCOZEB, OXYDEMETON-METHYL, PHORATE, TRIALLATE, TRIAZOPHOS.

**Other possibly hazardous pesticides used:** ALLOXYDIM-SODIUM, BROMOPHOS, CHLORFENVINPHOS, CHLORPROPHAM, COPPER HYDROXIDE, DALAPON, DIAZINON, DICLOFOP-METHYL, DI-1-P-MENTHENE, FENURON, FLUAZIFOP-P-BUTYL, LINURON, MALATHION, METALAXYL, METOXURON, PENTACHLOR, PIRIMICARB, PIRIMIPHOS-METHYL, PROMETRYN, PYRAZOPHOS, QUINALPHOS, SETHOXYDIM, TCA, THIABENDAZOLE, THIRAM, TRIADIMEFON.

**Parsnips** In the UK in 1988/9, 24 UK parsnip samples were tested for 15 different pesticides: none were found above reporting limits. Similar results were obtained in Sweden in 1989.

**Known 'nasty' pesticides used on or around parsnips:** ALDICARB, BENOMYL, CAPTAN, CARBOSULFAN, DIMETHOATE, DISULFOTON, DSM, MANCOZEB, PHORATE, THIRAM, TRIAZOPHOS.

**Ohter possibly hazardous pesticides used:** ALLOXYDIM-SODIUM, BROMOPHOS, CHLORFENVINPHOS, CHLORPROPHAM, COPPER HYDROXIDE, DALAPON, DIAZINON, DICLOFOP-METHYL, DI-1-P-MENTHENE, FENURON, FLUAZIFOP-P-BUTYL, LINURON, MALATHION, METALAXYL, METOXURON, PENTACHLOR, PIRIMICARB, PIRIMIPHOS-METHYL, PROMETRYN, PYRAZOPHOS, QUINALPHOS, SETHOXYDIM, TCA, THIABENDAZOLE, TRIADIMEFON.

**Passion fruit** In Sweden in 1989 samples of 3 imported batches were tested and no residues were found.

**Known 'nasty' pesticides used on or around passion fruit:** ACEPHATE, CARBARYL, DIAZINON, DICOFOL, DIMETHOATE, MANCOZEB, MANEB, NALED.

**Other possibly hazardous pesticides used:** COPPER OXYCHLORIDE, MALATHION, PIRIMIPHOS-METHYL, SULPHUR, TRICHLORFON.

**Peaches** Over 42 countries export peaches. The average American eats 10 lb of peaches per year.

In 1988/9 Canada found a consignment of US peaches to contain violative levels of quintozene\*\*. In 1988/9 Canada detected DMF and triforine in 2 of 20 samples of imported peaches.

In 1987 in Australia, residues of DDT, dicloran, malathion, parathion and dicofol were detected in peaches. In Sweden in 1989, 64 imported samples of peaches were tested and 24 revealed residues including acephate, azinphos-methyl, dicloran, methamidophos and pirimicarb.

In 1988 in the US 62% of 177 domestic peaches sampled contained pesticide residues but none over the US tolerance level. For fruit imported into the US figures were 51% (of 151 sampled) and under 1%. The NRDC found that dicloran, captan and carbaryl detected in peaches could be reduced by washing the fruit.

The EPA registers approximately 100 pesticides for use on peaches but the FDA routinely monitors for only 55% of them.

**Known 'nasty' pesticides used on or around peaches:** ACEPHATE, AMINOTRIAZOLE, AZINPHOS-METHYL, BENOMYL, CAPTAN, CARBARYL, CHLOROTHALONIL, CYPERMETHRIN, DICOFOL, ENDOSULFAN, DIAZINON, DIMETHOATE, DIURON, DSM, METHOMYL, METIRAM, OXYDEMETON-METHYL, PARAQUAT, PARATHION, PHOSMET, ZINEB.

**Other possibly hazardous pesticides used:** ASULAM, BORDEAUX MIXTURE, COPPER HYDROXIDE, COPPER OXYCHLORIDE, COPPER SULPHATE, CUFRANEB, CUPRIC AMMONIUM CARBONATE, 2,4-D, DICHLOBENIL, DICHLOFLUANID, FENVALERATE, FERBAM, HEPTENOPHOS, IPRODIONE, MALATHION, METHAMIDOPHOS, PENDIMETHALIN, PERMETHRIN, SETHOXYDIM, TAR OILS, TERBACIL, TETRADIFON, THIOPHANATE-METHYL, TRIFORINE, VINCLOZOLIN.

**Peanuts** *(see also Nuts)* In 1987, each American consumed on average almost $6^1/_2$ lb of shelled peanuts.

In the UK, of 30 samples of peanut butter analysed in 1987, at least 12 revealed isomers of HCH: 9 pesticide residues were tested for.

In Australia, residues of DDT, endosulfan, heptachlor, fenitrothion, malathion and pirimiphos-methyl were all detected in 1987.

The US EPA refused permission in 1990 for a number of southern states to use the insecticide pirimiphos-methyl on stored peanuts because of concern about the additional dietary exposure to children which might result.

**Known 'nasty' pesticides used on or around peanuts:** As field or forage crop in the US: ALDICARB, BENOMYL, CARBARYL, CARBOFURAN, CHLOROTHALONIL, CHLOROPICRIN, DISULFOTON, FONOFOS MANCOZEB, MONOCROTOPHOS, PHORATE. Elsewhere: ALDRIN, GAMMA-HCH, DDT, DIELDRIN, HEPTACHLOR.

**Other possibly hazardous pesticides used:** As field or forage crop in the US: ACEPHATE, CHLORPYRIFOS, DIAZINON, ETHOPROP, FENVALERATE, MALATHION, METHOMYL,

PROPARGITE, QUINTOZENE. Elsewhere: CHLORPYRIFOS, COPPER, COPPER HYDROXIDE, 1,3-DICHLOROPROPENE, ETHOPROP, FENAMIFOS, FENSULFOTHION, FENTIN HYDROXIDE, IPRODIONE, METALAXYL, METAM-SODIUM, PCNB, SULPHUR, THIOPHANATE-METHYL.

In Texas, integrated pest management has reduced pesticide use on peanuts by 81%.

**Pears** In 1989, each person in the UK consumed an average over $3^3/_4$ lb of fresh pears. Average US consumption is 6 lb per person.

In 1987/8 Canadians detected residues of azinphos-methyl, captan, cypermethrin, dicofol, captafol, dimethoate, iprodione, phosmet, parathion, ethion, fenvalerate, endosulfan and phosalone in pears although none were over Canadian MRLs. In the same year Canada found 1% of a sample of pears imported exceeded the MRL on DDT** and 1% exceeded the MRL on folpet**.

In 1989 in Sweden, some imported Italian pears were found to exceed Swedish MRLs on EBDCs** and other imports contained residues of chlorothalonil, carbendazim, methidathion, phosalone, parathion and thiabendazole.

In 1988 the US detained pears from one Chilean shipper because of one pesticide residue. In the same year in the US 39% of domestic fruit sampled contained pesticide residues but none over the US tolerance level. (The figure for pears imported into the US was 28%). The EPA registers 100 pesticides for the treatment of pears and the FDA can routinely only detect around 50% of those.

**Known 'nasty' pesticides used on or around pears:** AMINOTRIAZOLE, AZINPHOS-METHYL, BENOMYL, CAPTAN, CARBARYL, CARBENDAZIM, CYPERMETHRIN, DELTAMETHRIN, DICOFOL, DIMETHOATE, DSM, DSM-S, GAMMA-HCH, NICOTINE, O-DM, PHORATE, ZINEB.

**Other possibly hazardous pesticides used:** AMITRAZ, ASULAM, BORDEAUX MIXTURE, BUPIRIMATE, 2-CHLOROETHYLPHOSPHONIC ACID, CHLORPYRIFOS, COPPER HYDROXIDE, COPPER OXYCHLORIDE, COPPER SULPHATE, CUFRANEB, CYFLUTHIN, DALAPON, 2,4-DES, DICAMBA, DICHLOBENIL, DIFLUBENZURON, DITHIANON, DIURON, DODINE, DOFENTAZINE, FENARIMOL, FENITROTHION, FENVALERATE, FOSETYL-ALUMINIUM, GIBBERLINS, GLYPHOSATE, HEPTENOPHOS, ISOXABEN, MALATHION, MCPA, MECOPROP, MERCURIC OXIDE, METALAXYL, MYCLOBUTANIL, 1-NAPHTHYLACETIC ACID, NAPROPAMIDE, NITROTHAL-ISOPROPYL, NUARIMOL, OCTHILIONE, OXADIAZON, PACLOBUTRAZOL, PENCONAZOLE, PENDIMETHALIN, PENTANCHLOR, PERMETHRIN, PHOSALONE, PIRIMIPHOS-METHYL, PROPYZAMIDE, PYRAZOPHOS, PYRETHRINS, ROTENONE, SODIUM MONOCHLOROACETATE, SULPHUR, TAR OILS, TERBACIL, TETRADIFON, THIOPHANATE-METHYL, THIRAM, TRIADIMEFON, TRICHLORFON, TRICLOPYR, TRIFORINE, VINCLOZOLIN.

Californian growers have cut pesticide use by 30% through integrated pest management.

**Peas** In 1989 each person in the UK consumed on average 6.6 lb of fresh and frozen peas.

In the UK in 1988/9 samples of 34 UK peas in the pod were obtained and 11 pesticides tested for: none were found.

In 1986 and 1987, 22 samples of chickpeas were purchased from UK retail outlets and analysed for organochlorine and organophosphorous pesticide residues. 2 samples contained such residues; very low levels of gamma-HCH and tecnazene were detected. 5 samples of pigeon peas, when similarly analysed, proved positive in 4 cases. DDT and pirimiphos-methyl residues were detected. 9 samples of cowpeas and 1 of pea pulses proved free of the main groups of pesticide residues.

In Poland between 1986-88, residues of EBDCs were detected in green peas but none above MRLs.

Outside the UK many different types of peas are grown. In 1988 in the US the following were detained: Chinese pea pods from three Chinese shippers with three different pesticide residues recorded; snow peas from three Dominican shippers containing five different pesticide residues; snow peas from one Honduran shipper with one pesticide residue; snow peas from one Mexican shipper with one pesticide residue; sugar peas from one Mexican shipper containing one pesticide residue.

**Known 'nasty' pesticides used on or around peas:** ALDICARB, AZINPHOS-METHYL, BENOMYL, CAPTAN, CARBARYL, CARBENDAZIM, CHLOROTHALONIL, CHLORPYRIFOS, CYPERMETHRIN, DELTAMETHRIN, DIMETHOATE, DSM, DSM-S, GAMMA-HCH, PHORATE.

**Other possibly hazardous pesticides used:** ALLOXYDIM-SODIUM, BENTAZONE, BIFENTHRIN, CHLORMEQUAT, CHLORPROPHAM, CYFLUTHRIN, CYANAZINE, DICLOFOP-METHYL, DI-1-P-MENTHENE, DIQUAT, DRAZOXOLON, FENITROTHION, FENVALERATE, FOSETYL-ALUMINIUM, FLUAZIFOP-P-BUTYL, GLYPHOSATE, HEPTENPHOS, IPRODIONE, MALATHION, MCPA, MCPB, METALAXYL, OXAMYL, PENDIMETHALIN, PIRIMICARB, PROMETRYN, PROPHAM, SETHOXYDIM, SIMAZINE, TCA, TERBUTRYN, TERBUTHYLAZINE, THIABENDAZOLE, THIRAM, TRI-ALLATE, VINCLOZOLIN.

**Peel** (see Lemons, Oranges)

**Peppers** (protected) (also known as capsicums) In Poland between 1986-88 residues of pirimiphos-methyl, MBC, iprodione, pirimicarb and vinclozolin were detected in red peppers. In 1987

Denmark found some peppers imported from Spain exceeded Danish MRLs**.

In Sweden in 1989 some Spanish peppers also exceeded Swedish MRLs on chlorpyrifos, endosulfan, methamidophos, trichlorofin and pirmiphos-methyl**. 88 out of 219 samples contained residues including carbaryl, acephate, cypermethrin, diazinon, methamidophos, methidathion, omethoate, chlorfenson, pirimicarb and vinclozolin.

In 1988 the US detained peppers from one Chinese shipper for one pesticide residue; nine Dominican shippers for two pesticide residues; three Jamaican shippers for three pesticide residues and twenty Mexican shippers for seven different pesticide residues. In 1988 in the US, of 1,051 peppers sampled, 54% contained pesticide residues and 1% were over US tolerance levels**. The EPA has over 70 pesticides registered for use on bell peppers and the FDA can routinely only detect about 60% of them.

None of the residues identified by the NRDC on peppers could apparently be reduced by washing.

**Known 'nasty' pesticides used on or around peppers:** ACEPHATE, AZINPHOS-METHYL, CAPTAN, CARBARYL, CARBENDAZIM, CHLORPYRIFOS, CHLOROTHALONIL, CYPERMETHRIN, DICOFOL, DELTAMETHRIN, DEMETON, CARBOFURAN, ENDOSULFAN, METHOMYL, NALED, NICOTINE, PARATHION, ZINEB.

**Other possibly hazardous pesticides used:** ACEPHATE, COPPER SULPHATE, DIAZINON, DIFLUBENZURON, ETRIDIAZOLE, ETHION, FATTY ACIDS, FENVALERATE, HEPTENOPHOS, IPRODIONE, MALATHION, METHOXYCHLOR, OXAMYL, PERMETHRIN, PHOSPHAMIDON, PIRIMICARB, PROPAMOCARB HYDROCHLORIDE, QUINTOZENE, RESMETHRIN, TETRADIFON, TRICHLORFON, VINCLOZOLIN.

## Pheasant (see Fowl)

## Pigeon (see Fowl)

## Pineapples
In 1988 in the US none of 31 domestic pineapples sampled contained any pesticide residues. In 1988 the US detained pineapples from one Mexican shipper for one pesticide residue. Of 228 imported pineapples tested in the US in 1988, 30% contained pesticide residues. There have been reports that fruit imported into the US contains heptachlor/chlordane residues.

In 1987 dicloran was found in pineapples in Australia. In 1989 in Sweden some Colombian pineapples were found to exceed

Swedish MRLs on diazinon** and some Costa Rican and Honduran pineapples on carbendazim**.

**Known 'nasty' pesticides used on or around pineapples:** CAPTAFOL, CAPTAN, DIAZINON, DIMETHOATE, DIURON, ETHYLENE DIBROMIDE, METHYL BROMIDE, MIREX, PARAQUAT.

**Other possibly hazardous pesticides used:** AMETRYN, ATRAZINE, BROMACIL, DALAPON, DIMEFURON, FOSETYL-AL, MALATHION, METALAXYL, OXAMYL, TERBACIL, THIABENDAZOLE.

**Plums** In 1989, each person in the UK consumed on average almost 4 lb of fresh stone fruit.

In the UK in 1988/9 a sample of 15 UK plums and 26 imported plums was tested for 12 pesticides. The tests revealed the presence of phosalone in 2 samples, carbendazim in 2 samples of domestic fruit, and carbendazim in 2 lots of plums imported from the US.

In Sweden in 1989 samples of 29 imported and 7 batches of domestic plums revealed no residues.

In India residues of DDT and BHC have been detected in domestic plums.

In 1988 in the US 28% of 58 samples of domestic plums and prunes contained pesticide residues but none were over the US tolerance level. For fruit imported into the US the figures were 81% and 0%.

**Known 'nasty' pesticides used on or around plums:** AMINOTRIAZOLE, AZINPHOS-METHYL, CARBENDAZIM, CHLORPYRIFOS, CYPERMETHRIN, DELTAMETHRIN, DIMETHOATE, DSM, DSM-S, O-DM, OMETHOATE.

**Other possibly hazardous pesticides used:** ASULAM, AZINPHOS METHYL, BENODANIL, BORDEAUX MIXTURE, CLOFENTAZINE, CUFRANEB, CYFLUTHRIN, COPPER HYDROXIDE, COPPER OXYCHLORIDE, COPPER SULPHATE 2,4-DES, DIFLUNEZURON, FENITROTHION, GLYPHOSATE, ISOXABEN, MALATHION, NAPROMIDE, 1-NAPHTHYLACETIC ACID, OCTHILINE, PENDIMETHALIN, PENTANCHLOR, PHOSALONE, PIRIMICARB, PIRIMIPHOS-METHYL, PROPYZAMIDE, PYRETHRINS, SIMAZINE, SODIUM MONOCHLORACETATE, TAR OILS, TETRADIFON, VINCLOZOLIN.

## Pole beans *(see Beans)*

## Pommelo

**Known 'nasty' pesticide used on or around pommeloes:** CARBOSULFAN.

**Pork** In 1989, each person in the UK consumed on average over 10 lb of pork, almost 11 lb of uncooked bacon and ham and almost $1/2$ lb of pigs' liver. In 1987 the average American consumed over 59 lb of pork.

In 1988/9 a small number of samples of UK produced ham contained ppDDE and gamma-HCH as did some imports from the Netherlands and Denmark.

UK bacon produced residues of ppDDE in 2 samples, dieldrin in 1, gamma-HCH in 1 and HCB in 1 from 29 samples taken in 1988-9. Imports from Denmark showed 1 ppDDE residue from 19 samples and the Netherlands showed 1 ppDDE sample from 8 tested. UK porcine fat revealed residues in 1 case of gamma-HCH, 1 of ppDDT and 1 of diazinon in 23 samples tested.

In Yorkshire, England, in 1990 several hundred pigs from over 100 farms had to be slaughtered because they had apparently been adversely affected by eating contaminated food. The food contained the pesticide isofenphos, which is not licensed in the UK.

In 1988/9 Canada found 17% of the pigs' livers that it tested contained violative levels of pentachlorophenol**.

In Australia in 1987, DDT, dieldrin, chlorpyrifos-methyl, pirimiphos-methyl and fenitrothion were all detected in pork sausages.

**Known 'nasty' pesticides used on or around the pigs:** ALDRIN, CARBOPHENOTHION, CHLORDANE, CHLORPYRIFOS, DDT, DIAZINON, DICHLORVOS, DIELDRIN, ENDRIN, HCB, HEPTACHLOR, LINDANE, PHOSMET.

**Other possibly hazardous pesticides used:** AMITRAZ, BROMOPHOS, CHLORFENVINPHOS, COUMAPHOS, CROTOXYPHOS, DIOXATHION, FENTHION, FENVALERATE, IVERMECTIN, PERMETHRIN.

## Potatoes

The average Briton eats 118 lb of potatoes a year; the average American 79 lb.

In the UK in 1989, residues were detected in 8 out of 36 samples of new potatoes and 32 out of 57 main crop samples. Multiple residues were found in 11 out of 57 main crop potatoes analysed. Pesticides found included chlorpropham, dieldrin, tecnazene and thiabendazole on main crop; and dieldrin and tecnazene in new potatoes. Imported potatoes from Cyprus contained chlorpropham, dieldrin and ppDDE, tecnazene, thiabendazole and inorganic bromides; tecnazene was found in potatoes from Morocco and Spain.

In 1988 the US Food and Drugs Administration found 18% of the potatoes it sampled contained aldicarb residues. The highest level found was 0.71 parts per million and the EPA tolerance for aldicarb is 1 part per million (FDA *Residues Report,* 1988). In the same year in the US 23% of a sample of 30 imported potatoes contained pesticide residues. The EPA approves 90 pesticides for use on potatoes and the FDA can routinely detect only 55%. US potatoes still reveal residues of DDT, dieldrin and chlordane despite the fact that these chemicals were banned in 1978 for vegetable treatment. The NRDC reported DDT, chlorpropham, dieldrin, aldicarb and chlordane on US potatoes: of these only DDT was known to be reduced by washing.

In Sweden in 1989 some Belgian potatoes exceeded Swedish MRLs on thiabendazole** as did Canadian ones for chlorpropham** and UK ones for tecnazene**, thiabendazole** and chlorpropham**. In a sample of 139 imported potatoes, 27 contained residues including diquat.

In Poland between 1986-88 lindane and other HCH isomers were detected but only DSM exceeded Polish MRLs**.

**Known 'nasty' pesticides used on or around potatoes:** ALDICARB, AZINPHOS-METHYL, CARBARYL, CARBENDAZIM, CHLOROTHALONIL, CYPERMETHRIN, DELTAMETHRIN, DICOFOL, DIMETHOATE, DSM, DSM-S, FONOFOS, MANCOZEB, MANEB, NICOTINE, O-DM, TECNAZENE.

**Other possibly hazardous pesticides used:** CHLORPYRIFOS, CHLORFENVINPHOS, COPPER HYDROXIDE, COPPER SULPHATE, CYANAZINE, CYMOXANIL, DALAPON, 1,3-DICHLOROPROPENE, DICLOFOP-METHYL, DI-P-MENTHENE, DIQUAT, EBDC COMPLEX, EPTC, FENTIN ACETATE, FENTIN HYDROXIDE, FERBAM, HEPTENOPHOS, IMAZALIL, IPRODIONE, LINURON, MALATHION, MALEIC HYDRAZIDE, METALAXYL, METHAM-SODIUM, METRIBUZIN, METOXURON, MONOLINURON, OCTHILIONE, OXADIXYL, OXAMYL, PARAQUAT, PENCYCURON, PENDIMETHALIN, PIRIMICARB, POTASSIUM SORBATE, PROMETRYN, PYRETHRINS, SETHOXYDIM, SODIUM PROPIONATE, SODIUM METABISULPHATE, TCA, TERBUTRYN, THIABENDAZOLE, THIOFANOX, TOLCLOFOS-METHYL, TRIAZOPHOS, TRIETAZINE, ZINC, ZINC OXIDE.

## Poultry *(see also Fowl)* 

In the UK in 1988 average consumption of chicken was 24.4 lb per person. Average egg consumption was over 8.6 lb per person. Americans eat over 31 lb of eggs and over 62 lb of oven-ready chicken each per year.

In 1987 fenitrothion and DDT were detected in chickens in Australia.

In 1984/5, of 122 samples of UK chickens tested, 36 contained very low residue levels, including gamma-HCH, HCB and dieldrin. In the same period, one out of eight imported chickens contained very low levels of gamma-HCH.

Very low levels of some organo-chlorines (gamma-HCH) were detected in UK eggs in 1984-8. 12 out of 25 samples analysed in 1984/5 also contained very low levels of pentachlorophenol.

In 1988, 299 samples of US eggs and egg products were tested; 10% contained residues, but none contravened US regulations.

In India, eggs have been found to contain organo-chlorine residues including DDT, BHC, heptachlor and endrin.

**Known 'nasty' pesticides used on or around the birds:** CARBARYL, DICHLORVOS, DIMETHOATE, METHOMYL, NICOTINE.

**Other possibly hazardous pesticides which may be used:** FENVALERATE, MALATHION, PERMETHRIN, PETROLEUM OIL (CRUDE), PYRETHRINS.

## Prunes (see Plums)

## Pumpkins In the UK in 1986, 100% of a representative sample of the crop was found to have been treated with pesticidal seed treatments. In 1987 10 samples of pumpkin seed were analysed and 4 contained inorganic bromide.

In 1988 in the US pumpkins from one Costa Rican shipper were detained because of pesticide residues. Of 20 imported pumpkins sampled in the US in 1988, 10% contained pesticide residues but none over the US tolerance level.

In 1987 dicofol, dieldrin and heptachlor were all detected in pumpkins in Australia.

**Known 'nasty' pesticides used on or around pumpkins:** CARBARYL, ENDOSULFAN, PARATHION.

**Other possibly hazardous pesticides used:** ESFENVALERATE, FENVALERATE, MALATHION, METHOXYCHLOR, TRICHLORFON.

## Quinces In Sweden in 1989 residues of monocrotophos were detected in the one imported quince sample analysed.

**Known 'nasty' pesticides used on or around quinces:** AMINOTRIAZOLE, MONOCROTOPHOS.

## Rabbit In the UK in 1988/9, 13 samples of imported Chinese rabbit were found to contain various HCH isomers, 1 above the UK MRL**. In UK rabbits, 1 of a sample of 1 contained beta-HCH residues.

In 1984, a small survey of wild rabbits was carried out on the Scottish mainland and in Skye. 12 adult rabbits were analysed for pesticide residues and low levels of organochlrines including dieldrin and metabolites of DDT were found in the livers. No residues above the reporting limit at the time were detected in muscles. In 1985 and 1986, wild rabbits in Fife (Scotland) also contained low levels of dieldrin in the liver. No detailed studies exist which compare a wide range of pesticides likely to be found in either wild or commercially-reared rabbits in the UK today.

**Radicchio** In 1988 in the US 8% of a sample of 62 imported batches contained pesticide residues.

**Known 'nasty' pesticides used on or around radicchio:** DELTAMETHRIN, DIAZINON, DSM.

**Other possibly hazardous pesticides used:** IPRODIONE, MALATHION.

**Radishes** In the UK in 1986, 100% of a representative sample of radishes were treated with insecticides, 10% with fungicides and 100% with herbicides.

**Known 'nasty' pesticides used on or around radishes:** AZINPHOS-METHYL, CARBARYL, CARBENDAZIM, CHLOROTHALONIL, DIMETHOATE, ENDOSULFAN, MANEB, METHOMYL, METHYL-PARATHION, MEVINPHOS, NALED, PARATHION, ZINEB.

**Other possibly hazardous pesticides used:** CHLORPYRIFOS, DIAZINON, DISULFOTON, ESFENVALERATE, FENVALERATE, METHAMIDOPHOS, METHOXYCHLOR, METALAXYL, PERMETHRIN, ROTENONE, PCNB, TRICHLORFON.

**Raisins** *(see Grapes)*

**Raspberries** In Sweden in 1989, 1 sample of raspberries from Chile contained vinclozolin. In Poland between 1986-88 residues of dichlofluanid and iprodione were detected.

In the US in 1988, raspberries from two Chilean shippers were detained because of two different pesticide residues.

**Known 'nasty' pesticides used on or around raspberries:** ATRAZINE, AZINPHOS-METHYL, BENOMYL, CAPTAN, CARBARYL, CARBENDAZIM, CHLOROTHALONIL, CYPERMETHRIN, DELTAMETHRIN, DSM, DSM-SULPHONE, ENDOSULFAN, GAMMA-HCH, MANCOZEB, ODM, THIRAM.

**Other possibly hazardous pesticides used:** ASULAM, BENODANIL, BUPIRIMATE, BROMACIL, CHLORPYRIFOS, CHLORTHAL-DIMETHYL, COPPER OXYCHLORIDE, COPPER SULPHATE, CRESYLIC ACID, CUFRANEB, CUPRIC AMMONIUM, CYANAZINE, DALAPON, DICHLOBENIL,

DICHLOFLUANID, DIMETHOATE, 2,4-DES, FENARIMOL, FENITROTHION, HEPTENOPHOS, IPRO-DIONE, ISOXABEN, LENACIL, METALAXYL, MALATHION, NAPROPAMIDE, PARAQUAT, PEN-DIMETHALIN, PIRIMICARB, PROPYZAMIDE, PYRETHRINS, ROTENONE, SIMAZINE, TAR OILS, TRIADIMEFON, TRIFLURALIN.

## Rhubarb
In 1989 the average Briton consumed just under $3/4$ lb of fresh rhubarb.

In the UK in 1986, 33% of a representative sample of the crop had been treated with a herbicide.

**Known 'nasty' pesticides used on or around rhubarb:** CHLORPYRIFOS, CYPER-METHRIN, NICOTINE, TRIAZOPHOS.

**Other possibly hazardous pesticides used:** CHLORPROPHAM, DALAPON, 2,4-DES, FENURON, GIBBERLINS, PROPYZAMIDE, SIMAZINE, TCA.

## Rice
In 1989 the average Briton consumed just under $3^1/2$ lb of rice.

In the UK in 1988/9, rice samples of white long grain, brown long grain and white round grain were analysed. 2 samples of imported rice contained residues of pirimiphos-methyl and 1 of chlorpyrifos-methyl above MRL limits**. 12 samples of rice from Surinam exceeded the inorganic bromide MRLs**. 208 samples in all were analysed and of these 138 were analysed for inorganic bromide. The results included identification of residues of malathion in 3 cases, pirimiphos-methyl in 8, fenitrothion in 1 and ppDDT in 2. Italian rice contained malathion, pirimiphos-methyl, fenitrothion and inorganic bromides; US rice contained the first two chemicals as did rice from Surinam.

In 1987 pirimiphos-methyl residues were detected in rice in Australia.

In India residues of DDT and BHC have been detected in rice in the past.

In 1988 in the US 18% of domestic rice sampled for pesticides contained residues but only 1% contained violative residues. 5% of imported rice sampled contained pesticide residues but none violated US standards.

**Known 'nasty' pesticides used on or around rice:** ACEPHATE, BENOMYL, CAR-BARYL, CARBENDAZIM, CARBOFURAN, CHLORPYRIFOS, DIAZINON, ENDOSULFAN, MANCOZEB, MONOCROTOPHOS, NALED, OMETHOATE, TRIAZOPHOS.

**Other possibly hazardous pesticides used:** BIFENOX, BPMC 2,4-D, FENITROTHION, FENTHION, FURATHIOCARB, ISOPROCARB, ISOXATHION, MALATHION, OXADIAZON, PIRIMIPHOS-METHYL, PROPOXUR, TERBUFOS, THIOBENDICARB, TRICHLORFON.

Rice pests can be controlled by non-chemical means. The army worm and rice borer can be killed by raising the water levels in the paddy fields. This suffocates the army worm's eggs and drowns the larvae of the rice borer. In China, ducks are used to feed on pests in the paddy fields.

The striped borer, which attacks rice, can be deterred when resistant rice varieties are grown.

Integrated pest management has been successful in Asia and the Philippines.

## Runner beans (see Beans)

## Rye (see Cereals)

## Sesame
In the UK in 1988/9, of 10 samples of sesame seed tested, 5 contained inorganic bromide. Of 6 samples of crushed sesame seed spread (tahini), 3 contained alpha-HCH and 3 gamma-HCH.

**Known 'nasty' pesticides which may be used on or around sesame:** CARBOSULFAN, DICOFOL, ENDOSULFAN, METHOMYL, MONOCROTOPHOS, PARATHION-METHYL, TRIAZOPHOS.

**Other possibly hazardous pesticide used:** METHAMIDOPHOS.

## Sheep
In 1989, the average Briton consumed over 10 lb of mutton, lamb and lamb's liver. In 1987 the average American consumed 13 lb of mutton and lamb.

In the UK in 1988/9, 1 sample of lamb's kidney exceeded UK MRL for diazinon**. On 69 samples of imported lamb in the UK, 19 showed residues: of these isomers of HCH showed in New Zealand lamb as did diazinon. 4 samples of UK ewes' cheese produced residues of HCH isomers and dieldrin. 42 out of 44 imported samples of ewes' cheese also produced residues: these were mainly from France, Greece, Denmark and Cyprus.

In 1987 DDT was detected in lamb chops.

**Known 'nasty' pesticides used on or around sheep:** ALDRIN, CARBOPHENOTHION, CHLORDANE, CHLORPYRIFOS, DDT, DIAZINON, ENDRIN, GAMMA-HCH, HEPTACHLOR.

**Other possibly hazardous pesticides used:** BROMOPHOS, CHLORFENVINPHOS, COUMAPHOS, DELNAR, FENVALERATE, MALATHION, PROPETAMPHOS.

## Snap beans *(see Beans)*

## Sorrel

**Known 'nasty' pesticide used on or around sorrel:** DELTAMETHRIN.

## Soya beans *(see Beans)*

## Spices

In 1988 in the US, 52% of a sample of 21 imported ground spices contained pesticide residues, and of the sample 5% exceeded US tolerance levels**. 9% of a sample of 11 other imported spices contained pesticide residues.

In India pesticide residues detected in the past include DDT and BHC at very low levels in black pepper, celery seed, dill seed, fennel, ginger and turmeric.

## Spinach

In 1986 in the UK, 95% of a representative sample of the crop had been treated with insecticides and 95% with herbicides.

In Canada in 1988/9 there were particular concerns about EBDCs in spinach from the US and Mexico.

In 1988 in the US, 51% of a sample of 71 imported spinach plants contained pesticide residues and 4% of the sample exceeded US tolerance levels**. The EPA has 50 or more pesticides approved for use on spinach but can only routinely detect 55% of those residues.

The NRDC reported endosulfan, DDT, methomyl, methamidophos and dimethoate in spinach; only methomyl residues would be reduced by washing.

**Known 'nasty' pesticides used on or around spinach:** CARBARYL, CYPERMETHRIN, DIAZINON, DIMETHOATE, DSM, NICOTINE, THIRAM, ZINEB.

**Other possibly hazardous pesticides used:** CHLORPROPHAM, FENURON, HEPTENOPHOS, LENACIL, MALATHION, PIRIMICARB, PROPAMOCARB HYDROCHLORIDE, TRICHLORFON.

## Squashes

In 1988 the US detained squahses from 15 Dominican shippers with five different pesticide residues recorded; from one Guatemalan shipper with one pesticide residue; from three Mexican shippers with three different pesticide residues. In the same year 31% of squashes imported into the US, from a sample of 658, contained pesticide residues but none exceeded the US tolerance.

**Known 'nasty' pesticides used on or around squashes:** CARBARYL, CAR-BOFURAN, DIAZINON, ENDOSULFAN, METHOMYL, NALED.

**Other possibly hazardous pesticides used:** ESFENVALERATE, FENVALERATE, MALATHION, METHOXYCHLOR.

# Strawberries In the UK in 1988/9, 10 domestic and 11 imported samples of strawberries were tested for 23 pesticide residues. 1 sample of UK strawberries contained EBDCs above the UK MRL** and 1 sample contained multiple residues. Other residues detected on domestic samples were bupirimate, iprodione and vinclozolin. On imported fruit, there were residues of chlorothalonil from Spain, dichlofluanid from Israel, iprodione from Spain and vinclozolin from Spain.

In Sweden in 1989 some Belgian fruit exceeded Swedish MRLs on pirimicarb** as did Chilean fruit on EBDCs** and Spanish fruit on carbendazim**.

Cyrpus fruit has also shown residues above EC permitted levels on some strawberries**.

In 1988 the US detained strawberries from two Mexican shippers with two different pesticides detected. In 1990 the US reported finding dichlofluanid at levels between 0.01 and 3.29 parts per million on frozen strawberries imported from Poland. In the late 1980s the NRDC reported that more pesticide residues were detected on this fruit than in most fruit and vegetables. 86% of imported fruit had residues from 39 different pesticides. The EPA registers more than 70 pesticides for use on the fruit and the FDA can routinely monitor for the residues of approximately half of them.

Captan is the only pesticide whose residues can apparently be reduced by washing.

**Known 'nasty' pesticides used on or around strawberries:** ALDICARB, AZINPHOS-METHYL, BENOMYL, CAPTAN, CARBARYL, CHLOROTHALONIL, CYHEXATIN, DI-AZINON, DICOFOL, DIMETHOATE, DINOCAP, DINOSEB, DISULFOTON, DSM, ENDOSULFAN, GAMMA-HCH, NALED, METHOMYL, MEVINPHOS, NICOTINE, OD-M, PHORATE.

**Other possibly hazardous pesticides used:** ALLOXYDIM-SODIUM, ASULAM, BUPIRI-MATE, CARBOFURAN, CHLOROXURON, CLOPYRALID, COPPER OXYCHLORIDE, CYFLUTHRIN, 2,4-DES, 1,3-DICHLOROPROPEN, DIPHENAMID, DIQUAT, ETRIDIAZOLE, FENARIMOL, FEN-BUTATIN OXIDE, FENITROTHION, FENURON, FLUAZIFOP-P-BUTYL, FOSETYL-ALUMINIUM, HEP-TENOPHOS, IPRODIONE, LENACIL, MALATHION, MCPA, METALAXYL, NAPROPAMIDE,

PARAQUAT, PENDIMETHALIN, PENTANCHLOR, PHENMEDIPHAM, PIRIMICARB, PROPACHLOR, PROPAMOCARB HYDROCHLORIDE, PROPYZAMIDE, PYRETHRINS, SETHOXYDIM, SIMAZINE, SULPHUR, TERBACIL, TETRADIFON, THIRAM, TRIADIMEFON, TRIAZOPHOS, TRICHLORFON, TRIFLURALIN, VINCLOZOLIN.

## Sugar beet and cane sugar In 1988 the average Briton consumed 22½ lb of sugar.

**Known 'nasty' pesticides used on or around the produce:** Beet: BENOMYL. Cane: ALACHLOR, CHLORPYRIFOS, DIURON, PARAQUAT.

**Other possibly hazardous pesticides used:** Beet: CHLORIDAZON, ETHOFUMESATE, METALAXYL, METAMITRON, PHEMEDIPHAM, QUIAZLOFOP-ETHYL, THIABENDAZOLE. Cane: AMETRYN, ASULAM, ATRAZINE, 2,4-D, DALAPON, 2,4-DB, METRIBUZIN, PICLORAM, PROMETRYN, SIMAZINE, 2,4,5-T.

The beetle borer which attacks sugar cane has been controlled in Hawaii by the use of resistant varieties of sugar cane. Losses to the borer are also reduced if the cane is cut as early as possible.

## Sultanas *(see Grapes)*

## Sunflowers Of 10 samples of sunflower seeds tested in the UK in 1988-9, 7 contained inorganic bromide.

**Known 'nasty' pesticides used on or around sunflowers:** CARBOFURAN, CHLORPYRIFOS, CYPERMETHRIN, DELTAMETHRIN, FONOFOS, METHOMYL, MONOCROTOPHOS, TRIAZOPHOS.

**Other possibly hazardous pesticides used:** CHLORFLUAZURON, DIQUAT, ETHION, FENVALERATE, TEFLUBENZURON, TRIFLURALIN.

## Swedes In 1986 in the UK, 60% of a representative sample of crops had been treated with insecticides, 70% with pesticidal seed treatments, 4% with fungicides and 60% with herbicides.

**Known 'nasty' pesticides used on or around swedes:** AZINPHOS-METHYL, CARBARYL, CARBENDAZIM, CHLOROTHALONIL, DIMETHOATE, ENDOSULFAN, MANEB, METHOMYL, METHYL-PARATHION, MEVINPHOS, NALED, PARATHION, ZINEB.

**Other possibly hazardous pesticides used:** CHLORPYRIFOS, DIAZINON, DISULFOTON, ESFENVALERATE, FENVALERATE, METHAMIDOPHOS, METHOXYCHLOR, METALAXYL, PERMETHRIN, ROTENONE, PCNB, TRICHLORFON.

## Sweet-corn In the UK in 1986 34% of a representative sample of the crop had been treated with insecticides, 86% with pesticidal seed treatments and 100% with herbicides.

**Known 'nasty' pesticides used on or around sweet-corn:** ALACHLOR, AL-DICARB, CARBARYL, DIAZINON, DSM, GAMMA-HCH, METHOMYL, METHYL PARATHION, PHORATE.

**Other possibly hazardous pesticides used:** ATRAZINE, BENDIOCARB, CARBOFURAN, CHLORFENVINPHOS, CHLORPYRIFOS, CLOPYRALID, CYANAZINE, 2,4-DES, DIFENZOQUAT, ESFENVALERAT, FENITROTHION, FENVALERATE, PERMETHRIN, PYRIDATE, SIMAZINE, TERBUFOS, THIODICARB, THIRAM, TRIALLATE.

Integrated pest management has cut insecticide use on sweet-corn in Connecticut, USA, by up to half.

**Sweet potatoes** In 1988 in the US 10% of 21 imported sweet potato samples contained pesticide residues. The EPA approved over 40 pesticides for use on the crop but the FDA can routinely detect only 50% of these residues. The NRDC has reported residues of dicloran, phosmet, DDT, dieldrin and BHC on the crop, and only dicloran and DDT residues are known to be reduced by washing.

**Known 'nasty' pesticides used on or around sweet potatoes:** ACEPHATE, CARBARYL, CARBOSULFAN, CHLORPYRIFOS, DIAZINON, DICOFOL, ENDOSULFAN, LINDANE, MANCOZEB, TRIAZOPHOS.

**Other possibly hazardous pesticides used:** CHLORTHAL-DIMETHYL, DIPHENAMID, FENTIN ACETATE, FENVALERATE, MALATHION, METHOXYCHLOR, PYRETHRINS, TRICHLORFON.

The sweet potato weevil attacks the crop late in the growing cycle. An effective control method which does not require the use of expensive chemicals has been to harvest the crop as soon as it is mature, thereby significantly reducing weevil damage.

**Tahini** *(see Sesame)*

**Tea** In 1988 the average Briton consumed over $5^1/_4$ lb of tea.
In 87 samples of black tea analysed in the UK in 1987, 22 contained gamma-HCH, 13 other isomers of HCH, 1 dieldrin, 9 ethion, 2 cypermethrin and 3 fenvalerate: most residues were detected in Chinese and Indian imports.

**Known 'nasty' pesticides used on or around tea:** DIURON, PARAQUAT.

**Other possibly hazardous pesticides used:** AMETRYN, ATRAZINE, GLYPHOSATE, METRIBUZIN, SIMAZINE.

It is generally accepted that beverages are not an important source of pesticide residues in our diet. However, to protect tea workers and remove any possible problem for users, some pests of the tea plant can be controlled by non-chemical means. For instance, the shot-hole borer which is a tea pest in Sri Lanka can be controlled by fertilising crops better. This ensures good branch cover on the tea plant and this in turn reduces damage by the borer, which can get at less of the plant.

**Tomatillos** In 1988 the US detained tomatillos from 12 Mexican shippers because of four different pesticide residues detected in the vegetables. In the same year 63% of a sample of 162 imported tomatillos in the US contained pesticide residues.

**Tomatoes** In 1989, the average Briton consumed over 12$\frac{1}{2}$ lb of fresh tomatoes and over 4$\frac{1}{2}$ lb of canned or bottled tomatoes. The average American eats 24 lb of tomatoes a year.

53 different countries export tomatoes.

In 1983 and 1984, 21 of 101 samples obtained directly from UK growers contained pesticide residues: of these residues, 1 exceeded CAC or EC MRLs for DDT**.

In Sweden in 1989, of 113 domestic samples tested, 4 contained residues of vinclozolin, fenitrothion, quintozene and pentachloroanil. 15 of 325 imported tomatoes in Sweden contained pesticide residues which included chlorothalonil, endosulfan, inorganic bromides, carbendazim, chlorpyrifos, EBDCs, permethrin and methamidophos.

In Canada in 1988/9, residues of azinphos-methyl, captafol, chlorothalonil, chlorthal-dimethyl, diazinon, endosulfan, iprodione, permethrin, phorate and trichlorfon were detected in a sample of 97 domestic tomatoes.

In Poland between 1986-88, residues of EBDCs** above Polish MRLs and MBC, iprodione and vinclozolin were detected.

In 1988, the US detained tomatoes from one Venezuelan shipper with one pesticide residue detected. The EPA approves over 100 pesticides for use on the crop but the FDA can routinely measure the residues of only about 55%. The NRDC has reported the presence of residues of methamidophos, chlorpyrifos, chlorothalonil, permethrin and dimethoate on tomatoes; of these only chlorothalonil and permethrin can be reduced by washing.

In India in 1989, there were reports of DDT, lindane and BHC residues on tomatoes.

**Known 'nasty' pesticides used on or around tomatoes:** ALDICARB, AZINPHOS-METHYL, BENOMYL, CAPTAN, CARBARYL, CARBENDAZIM, CHLOROTHALONIL, CYPERMETHRIN, DIAZINON, DICOFOL, DIMETHOATE, DSM, ENDOSULFAN, GAMMA-HCH, MANEB, METHYL PARATHION, NICOTINE, ODM, TECNAZENE, ZINEB.

**Other possibly hazardous pesticides used:** BUPIRIMATE, CHLOROETHYL PHOSPONIC ACID, CLOPYRALID, COPPER OXYCHLORIDE, COPPER HYDROXIDE, COPPER SULPHATE, CUFRANEB, CUPRIC AMMONIUM CARBONATE, DICHLOFLUANID, DIFLUBENZURON, ESFENVALERATE, ETRIDIAZOLE, ETHANOL-IODINE, FATTY ACIDS, FENBUTATIN OXIDE, FENVALERATE, HEPTENOPHOS, IPRODIONE, MALATHION, METHAM-SODIUM, METHOXYCHLOR, METALAXYL, NABAM, OXAMYL, PEMETHRIN, PETROLEUM OIL, PENTANCHLOR, PHOSPHAMIDON, PIRIMICARB, PROPACHLOR, PROPAMOCARB HYDROCHLORIDE, PROPOXUR, PYRETHRINS, QUINTAZENE, RESMETHRIN, TETRADIFON, THIABENDAZOLE, THIRAM, TRICHLORFON, VINCLOZOLIN.

**Turnips** In 1989 the average Briton consumed over 3 lb of turnips.

In 1986 in the UK, 60% of turnips, in a representative sample, had been treated with insecticides, 70% with pesticidal soil treatments, 46% with fungicides and 60% with herbicides.

In 1988 in the US, 88% of a sample of 25 imported turnip greens contained pesticide residues and 16% of the sample exceeded US tolerance levels**. In the same year figures for imported turnips were 12% out of 17 samples.

**Known 'nasty' pesticides used on or around turnips:** AZINPHOS-METHYL, CARBARYL, CARBENDAZIM, CHLOROTHALONIL, DIMETHOATE, ENDOSULFAN, MANEB, METHOMYL, METHYL-PARATHION, MEVINPHOS, NALED, PARATHION, ZINEB.

**Other possibly hazardous pesticides used:** CHLORPYRIFOS, DIAZINON, DISULFOTON, ESFENVALERATE, FENVALERATE, METHAMIDOPHOS, METHOXYCHLOR, METALAXYL, PERMETHRIN, ROTENONE, PCNB, TRICHLORFON.

**Ugli** In Sweden in 1989 a sample of 2 imported uglis was taken and 1 contained pirimiphos-methyl.

**Urd beans** *(see Beans)*

**Venison** In the UK in 1988, 35 samples of deer kidney fat were tested for 14 different pesticide residues: none were detected.

**Water** In the 1980s in the UK atrazine, simazine, dimethoate, mecoprop, MCPA, NCPB, 2,4,5-T and 2,4-D have all been detected in water supplies. Persistent organochlorine pesticides like lindane have also been detected occasionally. In 1989, 298 UK water supplies were found to have been contaminated with pesticides exceeding EC legal limits. 16 different pesticides in the 298 water sources exceeded the EC legal limit and the total pesticide concentrations exceeded the EC limit in 76 cases**.

The UK Red List of Prescribed and Dangerous Substances and the EC lists, detailing those substances which should be tightly controlled because of water pollution problems, contain the following pesticides: gamma-HCH, aldrin, dieldrin, endrin, dichlorvos, atrazine, TBTO, trifluralin, fenitrothion, azinphosmethyl, malathion and endosulfan.

In the US in 1987, there were reports of pesticides polluting rain. In Ohio, 11 compounds were found in rainwater: alachlor, atrazine, metolachlor, DDT and atrazine all being recorded. In the US as long ago as 1979 aldicarb was found in wells used for drinking water which were near to fields where aldicarb had been used to treat potatoes. Cyazine, a pesticide linked to reproductive effects in animals, has also been found in US ground water.

In Italy in 1987, pesticide pollution of Italy's four richest regions occurred when Piedmont, Lombardy, Enilin and Romagna all exceeded EC limits for atrazine** in water supplies.

It is possible to measure some pesticides in water down to parts per billion (ppb). There are those who suggest that a pesticide present in water at 0.01 ppb often presents no threat to health or the environment. It is equally fair to point out that 0.1 millionth of a gram of dioxin causes tumours in mice and that coral cannot tolerate concentrations of the herbicide 2,4-D as low as 0.1 parts per million for as little as one day. Dioxins and 2,4-D are either pesticides or may be found in pesticides. Rainbow trout exposed to 38 parts per quadrillion of TCDD (a dioxin) in water over 28 days died in significant numbers a month later. A quadrillion is a million × a million × a million × a million!

Adverse reproductive effects of TCDD on rats, over three generations, at exposures of one part per trillion have also been noted.

**Water chestnuts** In 1988 in the US, out of 10 samples, no water chestnuts contained pesticide residues.

## Watercress

**Known 'nasty' pesticides used on or around watercress:** BENOMYL, DIMETHO-ATE, MANCOZEB.

**Other possibly hazardous pesticides used:** MALATHION, ZINC SULPHATE.

**Water melons** In Sweden in 1989, 2 samples of 15 imported water melons contained residues of acephate and chlorothalonil.

In the US only 4% of samples contained pesticide residues in the late 1980s, but in 1988, 8% of US water melons contained residues. Of 46 imported water melons sampled, 13% contained pesticide residues.

However, illegal use of aldicarb in California and Arizona in 1985 did result in residues on crops. In 1985 the illegal use of aldicarb on water melons was responsible for 638 probable pesticide poisoning cases and 344 possible cases in California. Figures for other western states and Canada totalled 333 probable and 149 possible. Levels in the melon which caused the poisoning ranged between 0.07 and 3 parts per million of aldicarb sulfoxide. These figures show how very low levels indeed of a pesticide or metabolite can cause poisoning in humans.

The EPA approves 30 pesticides for use on the melons and the FDA can identify about 50% of any such pesticides in routine residue tests. The NRDC reported residues of carbaryl, captan, methamidophos, chlorothalonil and dimethoate. Residues of chlorothalonil, captan and carbaryl can be reduced further by washing fruit.

**Known 'nasty' pesticides used on or around water melons:** AZINPHOS-METHYL, CAPTAN, CARBARYL, CARBOSULFAN, DICOFOL, DIMETHOATE, ENDOSULFAN, METH-OMYL, NALED, OXYDEMETON-METHYL.

**Other possibly hazardous pesticides used:** BENFURACARB, CHLORTHAL-DIMETHYL, DIAZINON, ESFENVALERATE, FENVALERATE, METHAMIDOPHOS, METHOMYL, METHOXYCHLOR, MEVINPHOS, PHOSPHAMIDON.

**Wheat** In 1988, the average Briton consumed the following amounts of bread and bread products: 50.5 lb of white standard loaves; 12.6 lb of wholewheat brown loaves; 14 lb of wholewheat wholemeal loaves; and 21 lb of other bread products including bread rolls. Figures for flour were 11.6 lb; for cakes 11.9 lb; for biscuits 17.6 lb.

In the UK in 1988/9, 15 of 58 samples of wheat germ contained residues of more than 1 organophosphorous pesticide: 16 samples contained no residues. Those pesticides identified included pirimiphos-methyl, chlorpyrifos-methyl, malathion, fenitrothion and etrimifos.

In 1987/8, 51% of a sample of Canadian domestic winter wheat contained tridemefon and 50% contained triadimenol.

Ethylene dibromide, a fumigant known to cause carcinogenic and reproductive effects in laboratory animals and used in the past in grain and bakery stores, was originally thought to be so volatile that it would not leave residues in food. In 1984 it was found in US grain and bakery products and was then phased out (Fan and Jackson 1989). This is another example of science policy getting it wrong on residues.

**Known 'nasty' pesticides used on or around wheat:** AMITROLE, BENOMYL, BROMOXYNIL, CARBENDAZIM, CHLOROTHALONIL, CHLORPYRIFOS, CYPERMETHRIN, DELTAMETHRIN, DSM, EBDCS, FONOFOS, GAMMA-HCH, IOXYNIL, MANCOZEB, MANEB, OMETHOATE, OXYDEMETON-METHYL, PARAQUAT, TRIAZOPHOS, ZINEB.

**Other possibly hazardous pesticides used:** BENODANIL, CHLORMEQUAT, CLOPYRALID, CYANAZINE, 2,4-D, DALAPON, DICAMBA, DICHLOBENIL, ETHIRIMOL, FENITHRONTHION, FENPROPIMORPH, FERBAM, FLUTRIAFOL, GLYPHOSATE, IMAZALIL, IPRODIONE, ISOPROTURON, LINURON, MCPA, MECOPROP, METOXURON, PENDIMETHALIN, PROPICONAZOLE, PROCHLORAZ, SIMAZINE, SULPHUR, TCA, TERBUTRYN, THIABENDAZOLE, THIOPHANATE-METHYL, THIRAM, TRIADIMENOL, TRIDEMORPH, TRIFORINE.

Pests and diseases can be controlled and greatly reduced on a variety of wheat crops using a range of techniques including climatic factors, mechanical means and biological controls.

Winter wheat can be protected from the stem-boring frit fly by late summer ploughing and then fallow which effectively controls the fly.

Wheat in Canada can be protected from the stem-boring sawfly by using trap crops of brome grass; the fly then lays its eggs on the grass and not the wheat and pest cannibalism results!

The planting of spring wheat avoids autumn aphids which bring with them the barleydwarf virus; winter wheat does not avoid this pest.

In Michigan, the cereal leaf beetle on wheat was defeated by growing wheat from pest-resistant varieties.

The hessian fly in the US was defeated, or at least curbed, by selecting pest-resistant varieties of wheat and careful planting times.

In India, early sowing of wheat freed crops from the attacks of the gall moth.

**Wine** *(see also Grapes)* In 1986 the average Briton drank over 11 litres of wine and the figure has been rising steadily. Alcohol is of course toxic itself as well as addictive, but people who drink organic wines do at least know what toxic substances they contain.

In the UK in 1987/8 residues were detected in a variety of wine samples. In 26 samples of red imported wine, methiocarb was detected in 2 samples and procymidine in 3. In 23 samples of white imported wine, iprodione was detected in 1 sample, methiocarb in 3 and procymidine in 2. In 5 samples of UK produced white wine, 1 contained iprodione, 1 procymidine and 1 vinclozolin. Multiple residues were detected in New Zealand red and white wine. Red and white Bulgarian, Italian and US wine did not reveal any residues.

In Canada in 1988/9 a small sample of domestic wine revealed detectable residues of azinphos-methyl, carbaryl, dimethoate and iprodione. Imported wine in Canada revealed residues of carbaryl and dimethoate.

**Yams** In 1988, the US detained yams from one Jamaican shipper because of one pesticide residue.

**Known 'nasty' pesticides used on or around yams:** BENOMYL, CAPTAN, CARBARYL, CARBOFURAN, DIAZINON, ETHYLENE, MANCOZEB, MANEB, METHYL BROMIDE.

**Other possibly hazardous pesticides used:** MALATHION, TRICHLORFON.

**Yoghurt** *(see Beef and dairy products)*

# PART 3
# The toxicity of pesticides

## HOW TO USE THIS SECTION

**PLEASE READ THESE NOTES BEFORE LOOKING AT THE FOLLOWING DATA.**

The data entries which follow provide short summaries of *some* of the information available on *some* of the pesticides listed in Part 2. They are not intended to be comprehensive.

- The information provided should give the reader an idea of the length of time a particular pesticide has been in use.
- The references to toxicity relate to the acute toxicity of the pesticide and will tell you how hazardous a pesticide is to those workers across the world who have to apply the chemicals.
- The categories of pesticides used are very broad ones. For instance certain chemicals control spiders and mites and are usually called acaricides and miticides. However for the sake of simplicity all these pesticides are grouped under the heading 'insecticides' here.
- References may be made to a pesticide being systemic, translocated or contact. Contact pesticides usually kill pests on the surface of a plant and so may usually but not always be more easily washed off produce. Systemic or translocated pesticides usually enter a plant or pest and therefore will not usually be washed off produce or removed easily by peeling.
- Details are given, where possible and where readily available, of

any residues found in food. This is not an exhaustive list and the entries in Part 2 may be fuller. A reference here to the detection of residues does not indicate that residue levels exceed national or international maximum residue levels. Consult Part 2 for these details. Most residues reported in this section are well below CAC, EEC and National MRL levels or do not have MRLs set for them in the UK. The significance of such levels and their indication of safe, dangerous or unknown effects on humans is discussed in Part 1 of this book.

● Some readers may wish to know, because of the wider environmental audit needs of pesticide hazard assessment, what the effects of the pesticides listed are or could be to wildlife, birds, bees and fish. Where possible, such potential effects are listed so that you can form some opinion not only about the effects of pesticides on workers, especially in agriculture in developing countries, but also of their potential effect on the wider environment and indeed the risks of disposal and penetration into water supplies.

● Information is given about which countries ban which pesticides for domestic use. Unfortunately, this does not necessarily prevent countries with bans from importing foods which may have been treated with those chemicals abroad.

● References to 'data gaps' in the following entries refer to gaps which exist in the information available on the toxicological effects of those pesticides listed.

## Main sources of information for this section

Board of Agriculture, National Research Council (1987), *Regulating Pesticides in Food,* National Academy Press, Washington DC.

EPA (1988), *Pesticides Fact Book,* Noyes Data Corporation, New Jersey.

FDA, Fact sheets and data summaries.

Hallenbeck W. H. and Cunningham-Burns, K. M. (1985), *Pesticides and Human Health,* Springer-Verlag, New York.

UNEP/IRPTC, Data files and literature reviews, Geneva.

UNEP, Lists of products banned or restricted (1984 and 1986).

Watterson, A. E. (1988). *Pesticide Users' Health and Safety Handbook: an International Guide,* Gower Technical Press, Aldershot.

# ABOUT THE PESTICIDES

**ACEPHATE:** potentially oncogenic insecticide used on citrus fruit in the US in the 1970s. Evidence of reproductive toxicity reported. Detected on corn in the US although that country does not permit its use on that crop.

**ADJUVANTS:** See 'Inerts' entry in this section.

**ALACHLOR:** potentially oncogenic herbicide used on soya beans and corn in the US since 1969. FDA could not detect this chemical in the 1980s through routine residue tests.

**ALDICARB:** carbamate insecticide, first registered in the US in 1970, with very high acute toxicity to workers and used on vegetables, peanuts, citrus fruit and potatoes. Data gaps existed in 1988 in residue studies. Very toxic to fish, wildlife and bees. Involved in cucumber poisoning cases in Canada and melon poisoning cases in the US in 1986. Netherlands has banned it from use in all catchment areas for drinking water supply. Contaminant in some US ground water. Banned in Israel in 1978. Prohibited for import into Philippines except in case of emergency.

**ALDRIN:** a persistent organo-chlorine insecticide. Potential oncogen and evidence of reproductive effects in laboratory animals. Banned in Sweden since 1970 because of its high acute toxicity and environmental impact. Banned in Portugal since 1986. Also banned in Turkey, Poland, Germany and the Philippines. Most uses of aldrin revoked in the UK by 1990 and all uses revoked by 1992.

**ALKYL MERCURY:** banned in Sweden since 1966 because of high toxicity and environmental impact.

**AMITRAZ:** potentially oncogenic insecticide used on cattle in the US since 1968. Widely used on pears in the US but it could not be detected by routine FDA residue tests in the 1980s. Registration of liquid formulation cancelled in Argentina in 1980. Harmful to fish.

**AMITROLE:** also known as aminotriazole, a residual herbicide first registered in the US in 1948. Banned in Sweden since 1972 because of carcinogenic risk to humans according to toxicological data. Banned in Finland in 1980 and withdrawn from Norway in 1982. Banned in Ecuador in 1985 because of health hazards. Not to be used on food crops in the US. Data gaps exist.

**ANTU:** a rodenticide banned in the Philippines. Withdrawn in UK in 1966 because of evidence that it and its impurities were potential carcinogens.

**ASULAM:** potentially oncogenic herbicide used on sugar cane since 1975 in the US and on vegetables and fruit in other countries.

**ATRAZINE:** potentially oncogenic triazine herbicide used on maize, sweetcorn and fruit. Banned in Sweden since 1989 due to its high mobility in the soil and potential for water contamination.

**AVERMECTIN:** an insecticide first registered in the US in 1986. US use allowed on non-crop land. High acute toxicity to workers. Very toxic to fish and birds.

**AZINPHOS-METHYL:** potentially oncogenic insecticide used on peaches and pome fruit and on fruit and brassicas in the UK. First registered in the US in 1956. Data gaps exist on this pesticide. Gaps on residue data existed in 1988. According to the EPA in 1985, residues appear to degrade fairly rapidly on crops but rates of residue decline vary widely depending on crops and environmental conditions. Cooking reduces residues but usage is on many crops which may be eaten raw. Dangerous to bees, fish and birds.

**BENAZOLIN:** systemic herbicide and growth regulator used on cereals. Harmful to fish.

**BENDIOCARB:** a carbamate insecticide used on sweetcorn, sugar beet and maize. Dangerous to fish and birds and toxic to bees.

**BENOMYL:** a confirmed animal oncogenic systemic fungicide used on vegetables and fruit and in the US since 1972 on citrus, rice, soya beans and stone fruit. Benomyl is the most widely used systemic fungicide in the world. Six formulations in 1982 based on benomyl and carbendazim were withdrawn in Sweden for home and garden use after evidence of genetic and foetal disturbances at high doses in laboratory animals, plus some evidence of increase in tumours in mice. Withdrawn in Finland in 1983 because of carcinogenic risks.

**BHC:** benzene hexachloride, an insecticide registered in the US in 1963 and used on rice and cotton worldwide. Evidence of carcinogenicity and reproductive toxicity. The US EPA banned it in 1978. Banned in Japan since 1971 and in Thailand. Dangerous to bees and harmful to fish.

**BINAPACRYL:** a fungicide and acaricide used on fruit and banned in the UK in 1987 on grounds of teratogenicity. Also banned in South Australia. Not approved for use in India in 1984. Still used in South Africa in 1988. Harmful to fish and livestock.

**BROMACIL:** a herbicide used on fruit in the US and banned in Sweden in 1990 due to its suspected carcinogenicity and mobility in soil. Evidence of thyroid abnormalities in animals. Dangerous to wildlife.

**BROMOPHOS:** an organophosphorous insecticide used on cabbages, fruit and vegetables. Some evidence of chronic effects on laboratory animals at high levels. Residues detected in apples, peaches, grapes and berries in USSR; residues persist on apples although washing reduces them by between 9% and 20%. Harmful to bees and dangerous to fish.

**BROMOXYNIL:** a contact herbicide known to cause deformities in laboratory animals but not generally detected on crops or in animal feed or forage. Harmful to fish and a wildlife hazard.

**BUPIRIMATE:** a systemic fungicide used on fruit and vegetables.

**CAPTAFOL:** potentially oncogenic fungicide first registered in the US in 1962 and used on apples, cherries and tomatoes. Data gaps existed on residue chemistry. Evidence of mutagenicity. Use restricted to pruning wounds in trees in Poland. Not permitted in East Germany, registration withdrawn in Norway and banned in Portugal since 1988. Very toxic to fish.

**CAPTAN:** potentially oncogenic fungicide first registered in the US in 1951 and used on almonds, apples, peaches and seeds and on fruit and vegetables. Evidence of mutagenicity and animal carcinogenicity. Restricted use in India. Severely restricted in Norway since 1981 because of potential carcinogenicity and high residues levels in edible crops. Data gaps exist on its residue chemistry. In Finland approval for its use was withdrawn in 1972 and later it was withdrawn in Sweden.

**CARBARYL:** a carbamate insecticide first registered in the US in 1958. Evidence exists on its mutagenicity and adverse chronic effects in animals. In India washing fruit and vegetables reduced its residues by between 66% and 86%; peeling by 96% and cooking by between 25% and 100%. Data gaps exist on its residue chemistry. Residues detected in apples and cows' milk in the USSR; and on plums and strawberries up to 30-35 days after treatment. Banned in Germany.

**CARBENDAZIM:** also known as MBC or methyl benzimidazole 2-yl-carbamate, a fungicide used widely on cereals, fruit and vegetables. Six formulations in 1982 based on benomyl and carbendazim were withdrawn in Sweden for home and garden use after evidence of genetic and foetal disturbances at high doses in laboratory animals plus some evidence of increase in tumours in mice.

**CARBOFURAN:** a systemic carbamate insecticide first registered in the US in 1969 and used on vegetables and other crops. Some evidence of reproductive effects in animals. One of its derivatives is mutagenic. Data gaps exist on its residue chemistry. Dangerous to fish, birds, wildlife and bees.

**CARBOPHENOTHION:** an organophosphorous insecticide used on cereals and other crops. Highly hazardous to people through acute effects, dangerous to wildlife. Data gaps include residue chemistry. Not approved for registration in India or in agriculture in East Germany.

**CARBOSULFAN:** a systemic carbamate insecticide used on fruit, rice and other vegetables. Not allowed for manufacture, sale or import in Malaysia since 1974. Dangerous to fish, birds and animals.

**CHLORDANE:** an organochlorine insecticide first registered in the US in 1948. Some evidence of oncogenicity in animals. Banned in Sweden in 1971 because of its persistence and environmental impact, and in Portugal since 1986. Also banned in Poland, Turkey and Germany. The EPA cancelled its agricultural use in 1978. Most uses of chlordane in the UK revoked in 1988 and all revoked by 1992. Data gaps existed in 1980s.

**CHLORDECONE:** an organochlorine insecticide withdrawn in the market in Sweden in 1978 because of its carcinogenic effect on laboratory animals and its persistent environmental impact. Not approved in Belgium because of its chronic toxicity. Not approved in Germany in 1978. Not registered in New Zealand.

**CHLORDIMEFORM:** potentially oncogenic insecticide used on cotton in the US. Banned in Turkey, Philippines and South Australia. Not used in India. Voluntarily withdrawn by the manufacturers in Cyprus in 1976 because of probable carcinogenicity. Voluntarily withdrawn from the US market.

**CHLORFENSON:** an organosulphur non-systemic insecticide used on fruit and vegetables. Linked to liver and thyroid effects in animals. In 1984 Singapore banned its import and sale for local use to safeguard water sources.

**CHLORFENVINPHOS:** an organophosphorous insecticide used on cereals, vegetables, rice and fruit. Some evidence of animal reproductive effects. Dangerous to fish and birds, toxic to bees.

**CHLORMEQUAT:** a growth regulator regarded as slightly hazardous. Used on wheat, oats, pears, tomatoes and winter rye.

**CHLOROBENZILATE:** potentially oncogenic insecticide and acaricide first registered in the US in 1953 and used on citrus fruit. Data gaps existed on the pesticide. Withdrawn in Sweden in 1979 because of its carcinogenic effect on laboratory animals, and in Finland in 1981. Banned in Ecuador, East Germany, New Zealand and Turkey. DDT may be a contaminant. Banned for local use in Singapore in 1984 because of water supply contamination risks.

**CHLOROPICRIN:** withdrawn in Sweden in 1966 because of its high acute toxicity, and banned in West Germany in 1988.

**CHLOROTHALONIL:** a fungicide first registered in the US in 1966 and used on vegetables, mushrooms, wheat and berries. Some evidence of animal carcinogenicity. Data gaps existed on residue chemistry. Dangerous to fish.

**CHLORPROPHAM:** a herbicide and growth regulator registered in the US in 1962 and used on potatoes and other vegetables and rhubarb. Evidence of animal mutagenicity, teratogenicity and carcinogenicity exists and there are also data gaps. Toxic to bees and should not be allowed to contaminate water.

**CHLORPYRIFOS:** an organophosphorous insecticide registered in the US in 1965 and used on fruit, vegetables and cereals. Data gaps exist including metabolism of the pesticide. Very toxic to birds and fish and dangerous to bees.

**CREOSOTE:** also known as tar oil, has been used as an animal dip. Banned in Swedish agriculture in 1986 due to suspected carcinogenicity.

**CYANAZINE:** a triazine herbicide first registered in the US in 1971 and used on cereals and vegetables. Some evidence of mutagenicity and reproductive effects in animals. Data gaps included residue chemistry. Harmful to fish.

**CYHEXATIN:** an insecticide registered in the US in 1972 and used on fruit, vegetables, hops and tomatoes. Evidence of birth defects and chronic effects in animals. Withdrawn in Sweden in 1972 due to foetal damage in laboratory animals even at low doses and skin penetration. No longer sold in New Zealand. Banned in Poland. Approval uses of cyhexatin revoked in UK in 1987. California suspended the use of the chemical in 1987.

**CYPERMETHRIN:** potentially oncogenic synthetic pyrethroid insecticide registered in the US since 1984 and used on cereals, fruit, vegetables, coffee. Some evidence of animal carcinogenicity. Highly toxic to fish and honey bees.

**DAMINOZIDE:** potentially oncogenic growth regulator, also known by its trade name 'Alar', used on apples and peanuts in the US since 1967 and not approved for use on food crops in New Zealand or Italy. Withdrawn by manufacturers in the US and UK by 1989.

**2,4-D:** potentially oncogenic phenoxyacetic acid herbicide first registered in the US in 1948 and used on wheat, rice, sugar cane and other crops. Some evidence of animal reproductive effects. Data gaps existed into the 1980s on its residue chemistry. Harmful to fish.

**2,4-DB:** a chlorophenoxyacetic acid herbicide used on cereals and other crops. Some evidence of embryotoxicity in animals. Harmful to fish.

**DALAPON:** a selective systemic herbicide used on vegetables including carrots and potatoes. Evidence of chronic animal toxicity. Residues have been found in asparagus, cereals and grapes, and trace elements have been found in cows' milk and hens' eggs. Avoid water contamination.

**DBCP:** or dibromochloropropane, a fumigant and insecticide. Evidence of animal carcinogenicity exists. Banned in Sweden in 1978 due to its damage to sperm. Banned in the Philippines. Colombia took action in 1982 to prohibit DBCP because of its health risks.

**DCPA:** a benzoic acid herbicide first registered in the US in 1958. Data gaps exist. Dermatitis evidence exists.

**ppDDE:** sometimes present in technical grade DDT and a breakdown product of DDT.

**DDT:** organochlorine insecticide registered in the US in 1945 and associated with animal carcinogenicity and reproductive toxicity. Banned in Sweden in 1975 due to its persistent environmental impact, in Portugal since 1974, in Finland since 1977, and in Thailand. The EPA cancelled all its uses in 1972. Also banned in Turkey and Poland. No longer used on food crops in New Zealand and all registrations cancelled there. Completely withdrawn in the UK in 1984 for environmental reasons.

**DELTAMETHRIN:** a synthetic pyrethroid insecticide used on cereals, vegetables, fruit and cattle which rapidly biodegrades. Very dangerous to fish and, in the laboratory, to bees.

**DEMETON:** organophosphorous insecticide registered in the US in 1949. Associated with birth defects and mutagenicity in the US. Data gaps existed through the 1980s on residue chemistry. Not approved for use in UK or USSR.

**DEMETON-S-METHYL:** organophosphorous insecticide used on fruit and vegetables. Some evidence of mutagenicity and reproductive effects in animals. Harmful to bees, birds, fish and animals. Apparently prohibited for use in USSR agriculture.

**DIALLATE:** potentially oncogenic herbicide used on sugar beets in the US since 1969. Evidence of animal carcinogenicity and mutagenicity. Harmful to fish. Banned in South Australia.

**DIAZINON:** an organophosphorous insecticide first registered in the US in 1952 and used on fruit and vegetables. Evidence of neurological effects and mutagenicity in animals. Very toxic to birds, dangerous to bees and harmful to fish.

**DICAMBA:** a translocated herbicide registered in the US in 1967 and used on corn, grain, sugar cane and asparagus. It may apparently be contaminated with nitrosamines. Possible evidence of mutagenicity. Data gaps existed in 1980s on residue chemistry. Harmful to fish.

**DICHLOBENIL:** a herbicide first registered in the US in 1984 and used on a range of food crops. Data gaps existed in the 1980s on its oncogenicity and residue chemistry. Some evidence of chronic effects on the liver and kidneys in animals.

**DICHLOFLUANID:** a fungicide used on fruit and some vegetables. Some evidence of mutagenicity. Harmful to fish.

**1,3-DICHLOROPROPENE:** banned in Sweden in 1988 due to its suspected carcinogenic effect and its high mobility in the soil.

**1,2-DICHLOROBENZENE:** banned in Sweden in 1984 because of its persistent mutagenic effects on laboratory animals.

**DICHLORVOS:** an organophosphorous insecticide used on fruit, vegetables and cattle. Evidence of mutagenicity and carcinogenicity. Data gaps. Acute hazard to bees and birds. Residues detected in fish sold for human consumption. According to USSR data, dichlorvos residues rapidly decline in food and fruit processing; washing, canning and juice making rapidly reduce residues down to zero levels.

**DICLOFOP-METHYL:** potentially oncogenic herbicide used on soya beans in the US since 1980 and on other vegetables and cereals. Toxic to fish.

**DICLORAN:** a fungicide registered in the US in 1961 and used on fruit and vegetables. Data gaps. Some evidence of chronic effects in animals. Harmful to wildlife.

**DICOFOL:** potentially oncogenic organochlorine insecticide used on citrus fruit and cotton and first registered in the US in 1957. Some evidence of carcinogenicity and mutagenicity in animals. Data gaps existed in the 1980s on residue chemistry. Toxic to fish.

**DICROTOPHOS:** organophosphorous insecticide used on coffee, citrus fruit and rice. Some evidence of mutagenicity and reproductive effects in animals. Not approved for use in UK and banned in Malaysia and East Germany. Very toxic to bees.

**DIELDRIN:** an organochlorine insecticide registered in the US in 1949 and associated with carcinogenicity, birth defects and reproductive toxicity in animals. Banned in Sweden in 1969 because of its high acute toxicity and environmental impact. The US cancelled all its use in 1974. Also banned in Turkey, Poland and Philippines. No longer used on food crops in New Zealand and all registrations cancelled there. All UK uses of dieldrin revoked in 1989.

**DIFLUBENZURON:** a urea-based insecticide first registered in the US in 1978 and used on soya beans and other crops. Some data gaps existed in 1980s on residue chemistry. Some evidence of reproductive effects and carcinogenicity in animals exists.

**DIMETHOATE:** an organophosphorous insecticide registered in the US in 1963 and used on corn, wheat, tea, rice, fruit and vegetables. Associated with carcinogenicity, birth defects, reproductive toxicity and mutagenicity in animals. Residues have been found in vegetables and fruit in the USSR in grapes, peaches, apples, cherries, plums, dried apricots, tomatoes and aubergines 2 months after treatment. Highly toxic to bees, harmful to fish and birds.

**DINOCAP:** a fungicide and acaricide used on fruit, vines and vegetables. Banned in Sweden in 1989 due to teratogenicity. Evidence of animal oncogenicity. Dangerous to fish.

**DINOSEB:** a contact herbicide and insecticide, also a growth regulator used on cereals, vegetables and fruit. Banned in Sweden in 1971 because of its high acute toxicity, in Ecuador in 1985 because of toxicity and in Poland, Norway, Thailand, Finland since 1987, and South Australia. Banned in the UK in 1987 on grounds of its teratogenicity.

**DIOXATHION:** an organophosphorous insecticide used on animal parasites and fruit. Not approved for agricultural use in UK but approved as an animal medicine. High acute toxicity to workers.

**DIPHENYLAMINE:** a plant growth regulator and insecticide registered in the US in 1962. Evidence of chronic effects in animals. Data gaps.

**DIQUAT:** a contact herbicide and desiccant. Some evidence of adverse animal effects at high doses and reproductive effect and mutagenicity data exist. Residues have been detected in rice and tolerances have been set for residues in US crops.

**DISULFOTON:** a systemic organophosphorous insecticide used on vegetables. Very toxic. Toxic to bees and dangerous to fish, birds and animals.

**DITHIANON:** a fungicide used on fruit, grapes, hops and coffee. Harmful to fish and toxic to bees.

**DITHIOCARBAMATES:** This group includes thiram and the EBDCs (ethylene bisdithiocarbamates) which are maneb, ziram, mancozeb, metiram and zineb. Since 1977, treatment of edible parts of plants in Sweden by mancozeb, maneb, propineb, thiram, zineb and ziram not allowed. With some crops like spinach, carrots and potatoes treated with EBDCs, high levels of ETU (see below) can be detected after cooking. Some evidence exists of reproductive effects and oncogenicity in animals. Data gaps existed on these pesticides in the 1980s.

**DIURON:** a urea-based herbicide used on fruit, sugar cane, pineapple and other crops. Residues have been detected in some fruit and vegetables. Some animal evidence on its carcinogenicity at high doses and reproductive effects. Harmful to fish. Data gaps existed in 1980s.

**DNOC:** a nitrophenol insecticide and desiccant used on fruit, cereals and vegetables. Highly hazardous. Toxic to bees and fish. Revoked in the UK in 1988 and 1989.

**DSM:** abbreviation for demeton-s-methyl (see above).

**EBDCs (Ethylenebisdithiocarbamates):** this group of fungicides makes up 57% of the total fungicide use worldwide. EBDCs can break down into ETU (qv) on cooking or food processing. ETU and EBDCs have been linked in animals with liver, lung and thyroid tumours, mutagenicity and birth defects. Residues have been detected in lettuces in France and approximately one third of all US fruit and vegetables are treated with EBDCs.

**ENDOSULFAN:** an organochlorine insecticide registered in the US in the early 1960s and used on rice, fruit and hops. Chronic effects in animals on liver and kidneys have been detected and there is some evidence of mutagenicity and animal carcinogenicity. Very toxic to fish. In India it has been found that washing fruit and vegetables reduced its residues by between 29% and 100% and cooking by 25% to 60%. Banned in Bulgaria, restricted in Denmark, Sweden, Finland, India and Thailand. Very toxic to fish and harmful to bees. Residues detected in celery, lettuce, spinach and strawberries and in water in several parts of the world, including the Americas and Europe.

**ENDRIN:** an organochlorine insecticide used on maize, sugar cane, rice and fruit. Some evidence of carcinogenicity, mutagenicity and reproductive effects in animals exists. Banned in Sweden since 1966 because of its high acute toxicity and environmental impact, and in Portugal in 1986. Also banned in Turkey, New

Zealand, Philippines, Finland since 1979, and Thailand. With-drawn in the UK. Toxic to fish, bees and very toxic to wildlife.

**EPN:** or 0-ethyl 0-4-nitrophenyl phenylphosphenollioate. This is an organophosphorous insecticide. Banned in the Philippines.

**ETACONAZOLE:** banned in Poland.

**ETHAFLURALIN:** potentially oncogenic herbicide used in the US on soya beans since 1982.

**ETHION:** an organophosphorous insecticide registered in the US in 1972 and used on apples, citrus fruit and cattle and other crops. Data gaps exist and data also under review. Toxic to fish and bees.

**ETHOXYQUIN:** a fungicide and plant growth regulator regarded as slightly hazardous.

**ETHYLENE DIBROMIDE (EDB):** a fumigant banned in Philippines. Withdrawn in the UK in 1981 as a grain fumigant because of its potential carcinogenicity. The EPA cancelled its use in the US in 1984. Prohibited for use in Chile in 1985 as a fumigant on fruit and vegetables.

**ETHYLENE OXIDE:** potentially oncogenic bactericide used on spices and walnuts in the US. Banned in Poland and prohibited for use in Germany in 1980.

**ETHYL PARATHION:** phased out in India. The non-official name for parathion (see below).

**ETU (Ethylene thiourea):** a metabolite of the EBDCs which may increase in the storage, processing and cooking of food treated with EBDCs. An animal teratogen and known to cause thyroid tumours in animals.

**FENITROTHION:** an organophosphorous contact insecticide used on fruit, tea, rice and cereals. Can react with other pesticides to make them more toxic. In India it has been found that washing fruit and vegetables can reduce residues by 17% and peeling by 9%. In the USSR it was found that residues declined on treated cherries and were not detectable after 10 days; on wheat it was 8 days and on potatoes it was 20 days. Dangerous to bees and harmful to fish and birds.

**FENPROPIMORPH:** a systemic fungicide used on cereals. Dangerous to fish.

**FENSON:** an insecticide. Import and local use banned in Singapore because of the need to safeguard water supplies in 1984.

**FENTHION:** an organophosphorous insecticide of moderate toxicity used on fruit, beet, rice and cattle. Residues have been detected in plants and water.

**FENVALERATE:** a pyrethroid insecticide registered in the US in 1972. Data under review.

**FLUAZIFOP-BUTYL:** a translocated herbicide used on vegetables. Harmful to fish.

**FOLPET:** potentially oncogenic fungicide used on pineapples in the US since 1983. Evidence of mutagenicity and reproductive effects in animals. Banned in Germany. Not approved for use in the UK, or Finland since 1972 because of toxicity. Banned in South Australia. Toxic to fish.

**FONOFOS:** an organophosphorous insecticide used on vegetables and seeds. Extremely toxic. Not permitted for use in East Germany and banned in Malaysia in 1974 because of toxicity and the availability of less toxic substitutes. Dangerous to fish and birds and toxic to bees.

**FOSETYL-AL:** an organophosphorous fungicide used on hops and pineapples with evidence of weak oncogenicity.

**GAMMA-HCH:** see lindane entry.

**GLYPHOSATE:** potentially oncogenic translocated herbicide used on hay and orchard crops in the US since 1976. Harmful to fish. Data gaps existed throughout the 1980s.

**HCB:** see hexachlorobenzene.

**HCH (benzene hexachloride or BHC):** Mixed isomers. Banned in Turkey, Poland and Philippines (as HCH/BHC), Cyprus in 1980, Ecuador in 1985, and Portugal in 1986. See BHC entry above.

**HEPTACHLOR:** an organochlorine insecticide which is persistent in the environment and is a known mouse carcinogen. Banned in Turkey and Philippines.

**HEXACHLOROBENZENE:** an organochlorine fungicide widely used on a variety of crops in the past. Evidence of mutagenicity and carcinogenicity in animals exists. Pentachlorophenol is the primary metabolite of this pesticide. Withdrawn in Sweden in 1980 because of its carcinogenic effects on laboratory animals and its persistence. Banned in West Germany in 1977, prohibited in Belgium and Denmark and banned in Portugal in 1986. Withdrawn in the UK in 1975 for environmental rather than human safety reasons.

**IMAZALIL:** a systemic fungicide used on cereals, fruit, vegetables and seeds. Some reproductive effects in animals reported. Residues reported in cucumbers. Water should not be contaminated with imazalil. Harmful to fish and bees.

**IMAZAPYR:** a translocated herbicide. Do not contaminate water.

**INERTS:** a general name for the adjuvants, solvents, stabilizers and other additives in pesticides in addition to the active ingredient. The EPA has a list of 1,200 inerts used in pesticide production, of which 50 are linked to adverse health effects, 300 are viewed as innocuous and approximately 800 have no information available on their health effects.

**INORGANIC BROMIDES:** Low levels of bromide occur naturally in nuts but higher levels come mainly from the use of the fumigant methyl bromide (see below).

**IOXYNIL:** a benzonitrile contact herbicide used on cereals, leeks, onions and sugar cane. Some evidence of thyroid tumours in animals, reproductive effects and mutagenicity. Banned in Poland. Not approved for garden use in the UK.

**IPRODIONE:** a fungicide registered in the US in 1980 and used on cereals, fruit, vines and vegetables. Chronic effects recorded in animals at high doses. Evidence of mutagenicity, liver, urinary and reproductive effects and immunological damage in animals. Harmful to fish.

**ISOCARBAMID:** a selective herbicide used on sugar beet and fodder beet. Banned in Poland.

**ISOPROTURON:** a urea-based contact and residual herbicide used on barley, rye and wheat.

**KELEVAN:** an insecticide, banned in Poland, and not marketed in Portugal because of its environmental and toxicological effects. Not cleared for use in the UK.

**KEPONE:** also known as chlordecone, and not approved for use in UK agriculture. An insecticide with evidence of carcinogenicity, mutagenicity and adverse reproductive effects attached to it.

**LEPTOPHOS:** an organophosphorous insecticide linked to adverse neurological effects in animals. Banned in the Philippines.

**LINDANE:** potentially oncogenic insecticide used on avocados and pecans. Registered in the US since 1955. Lindane has been detected on US corn even though it is not permitted for use on that crop. Banned in Sweden since 1988 because of its suspected carcinogenic properties and its persistence. No longer used on food crops in New Zealand where all registrations have been cancelled. Restricted use only to seed treatments in Poland.

**LINURON:** potentially oncogenic herbicide used on soya beans, vegetables and cereals. Registered in the US since 1966. Some evidence of animal carcinogenicity. Harmful to fish.

**MALATHION:** also known as mercaptothion, an organophosphorous insecticide registered in the US in the 1950s and used on a wide range of fruit and vegetables. Some evidence of reproductive effects in animals at very high doses and mutagenicity. In India it was found that washing fruit and vegetables reduced malathion residues by between 40% and 100% and cooking by up to 80%. Highly toxic to bees and harmful to fish.

**MALEIC HYDRAZIDE:** potentially oncogenic growth regulator used on onions and potatoes and registered in the US since 1955. Some evidence of animal carcinogenicity associated with impurities. Controlled in Guatemala because of potential carcinogenicity. Residues detected in onions and potatoes in the past.

**MANCOZEB:** potentially oncogenic fungicide used on fruit, small grains and vegetables and registered in US since 1962. ETU (qv) residues detected in treated crops. Harmful to fish. (See EBDCs above).

**MANEB:** potentially oncogenic fungicide used on fruit and small grains in the US since 1957 and with restricted use as a pesticide in Poland. Prohibited use in USSR. Residues detected in tomatoes and potatoes. Toxic to fish. (See EBDCs above).

**MBC or methyl benzimidazol-2-ylcarbamate:** another term for carbendazim (qv).

**MCPA:** a phenoxyacetic acid herbicide used on cereals and asparagus. Some evidence of weak mutagenicity and reproductive effects in animals. Harmful to livestock. Trace amounts detected in water in the US and Canada. In 1960s very low levels of residues were detected in food in the US. Data gaps existed in the 1980s.

**MECOPROP:** a systemic phenoxyacetic acid herbicide used on cereals and fruit. Some evidence of mutagenicity and reproductive effects in animals.

**MEFLUIDIDE:** a plant growth regulator and herbicide used on soya beans and other crops. Do not contaminate water.

**MEPIQUAT CHLORIDE:** a plant growth regulator used on barley. Harmful to fish.

**MERCURY:** banned in Turkey. Mercuric fungicides are also banned in Turkey. Mercury derivatives are banned in Poland. Mercuric chloride withdrawn in UK in 1965 on toxicity grounds. Mercury(11) chloride withdrawn in UK. Methyl mercury withdrawn in UK in 1971 on environmental grounds.

**METALAXYL:** a systemic fungicide used on hops, fruit, maize and vegetables. Some evidence of animal oncogenicity exists. Harmful to fish.

**METAMITRON:** a triazine herbicide used on sugar beet and other crops which should not be allowed to contaminate water.

**METHAMIDOPHOS:** a highly toxic organophosphorous insecticide first registered in the US in 1963. Data gaps exist and data is under review.

**METHIDATHION:** an organophosphorous insecticide first registered in the US in 1972 and used on field crops and fruit. Highly hazardous. Some evidence of oncogenicity exists and of reproductive damage at high levels in animals. Dangerous to fish and harmful to animals, birds and bees. Not approved for use in the UK. Too hazardous for general use in the Philippines except on bananas.

**METHOMYL:** potentially oncogenic insecticide with toxic metabolite (acetamide) used on citrus fruit, cotton and vegetables and registered in the US since 1963. Some evidence of chronic effects in animals exists and also mutagenicity. Banned in Malaysia in 1974. Dangerous to fish, bees and wildlife.

**METHOXYCHLOR:** an organochlorine insecticide used on a wide range of crops. Some evidence exists of carcinogenicity and reproductive effects in animals. Banned in Singapore in 1984 to safeguard water supplies.

**2-METHOXYETHYL-MERCURY ACETATE:** severely restricted in Sweden in 1979 and banned in 1988 as a seed dressing because of its high acute toxicity to workers, animals and its persistence in the environment.

**METHYL BROMIDE:** a fumigant, herbicide and fungicide first registered in the US in 1961 and widely used on nuts and other crops. Linked to mutagenicity, carcinogenicity and reproductive effects in animals.

**METHYL PARATHION:** an organophosphorous insecticide first registered in the US in 1954. Data gaps existed in 1980s and there is some evidence of carcinogenicity, reproductive effects and chronic effects in animals. Not approved for use in the UK and banned in Japan since 1971.

**METIRAM:** potentially oncogenic fungicide used on fruit and small grains in the US since 1967. (See EBDCs above).

**METOLACHLOR:** potentially oncogenic herbicide used on corn and soya beans in the US since 1976.

**METOXURON:** a urea translocated herbicide used on cereals and vegetables. Banned in Sweden in 1990 due to suspected carcinogenicity. Moderately toxic to fish.

**MEVINPHOS:** an organophosphorous systemic insecticide first registered in the US in 1958 and used on fruit and vegetables. Some evidence of mutagenicity exists. Dangerous to fish, bees, wild animals and birds.

**MONOCROTOPHOS:** an organophosphorous insecticide used on sugar cane, vegetables and peanuts. Highly hazardous to workers. Some evidence of mutagenicity exists. In India it was found that washing reduced residues by between 18% and 31%. Not cleared for use in UK. Very toxic to birds, shrimps, crabs and bees.

**MONOLINURON:** a urea based herbicide used on potatoes, leeks, vines and beans. Some evidence of reproductive effects in animals exists.

**MONURON:** a urea herbicide used on a wide variety of fruit crops. Some evidence of animal carcinogenicity exists. Withdrawn in Sweden because of its carcinogenic and mutagenic effect on laboratory animals in 1974 and 1988. Residues detected in citrus fruit in the USSR at low levels. Monuron and atrazine together increase their toxicity.

**NITROFEN:** a herbicide used on cereals and vegetables. Evidence of animal carcinogenicity and reproductive effects. Banned in Portugal, Finland, South Australia, Philippines and Cyprus and withdrawn in Canada, Denmark, New Zealand and Japan. Banned in Sweden in 1979 because of its teratogenic and carcinogenic effects on laboratory animals. Withdrawn in the UK in 1981 on grounds of mutagenic, carcinogenic and teratogenic hazard.

**ODM:** see oxydemeton-methyl.

**OMETHOATE:** a moderate to highly toxic organophosphorous insecticide not allowed for use in Malaysia since 1974 because of its toxicity and the availability of safer alternatives.

**OXADIAZON:** a herbicide used on rice, vines and fruit. Potentially oncogenic. Dangerous to fish and toxic to bees.

**OXAMYL:** a systemic carbamate insecticide used on vegetables and field crops. Highly hazardous. Dangerous to fish, birds, bees and wildlife.

**OXYCARBOXIN:** a fungicide used on cereals and vegetables. Some evidence of mutagenicity exists. Banned in Finland because of insufficient documentation. Dangerous to fish.

**OXYDEMETON-METHYL:** an organophosphorous insecticide. In India it has been found that washing fruit and vegetables reduces residues by between 18% and 22%. High acute toxicity to humans.

**PARAQUAT DICHLORIDE:** a potentially oncogenic herbicide and desiccant used on rice and soya beans in the US since 1961. Evidence of reproductive effects in animals exists. Banned in Sweden in 1983 because of the high acute toxicity and irreversible effects. Banned in Finland in 1985 because of acute toxicity. In the Philippines paraquat was considered too hazardous for general use and was restricted to institutional use on banana plantations only. Harmful to animals.

**PARATHION:** potentially oncogenic organophosphorous insecticide used on citrus and cotton and registered in the US since 1955 and also more generally on fruit, vegetables and nuts. Mutagenicity data exists. Extremely hazardous. Banned in Sweden in 1971 because of its high acute toxicity. Not approved for use in the UK. Parathion is banned in the Philippines. In 1984 one commentator estimated that the majority of the 500,000 pesticide poisoning cases occurring each year and the 20,000 pesticide-related deaths (WHO estimates) were due to parathion exposure. Extremely toxic to animals and toxic to fish and bees.

**PCNB:** potentially oncogenic fungicide used on cotton, peanuts and vegetables in the US since 1955.

**PENDIMETHALIN:** a herbicide used on cereals, vegetables, rice and fruit. Some evidence of liver damage in animal studies. Dangerous to fish.

**PENTACHLOROPHENOL:** a fungicide which has been used on cereals and in mushroom houses. Evidence of mutagenicity and reproductive effects in animals exists. Banned in Sweden in 1978 and 1982 because of highly toxic impurities and combustion products. Dangerous to fish.

**PERMETHRIN:** synthetic pyrethroid insecticide used on vegetables and fruit and first registered in the US in 1978. Evidence of reproductive toxicity in animals exists and some evidence of weak oncogenicity in mice and rats. Residues are primarily surface residues and they have been detected on lettuce, cabbage, peas and tomatoes. Dangerous to bees and extremely dangerous to fish.

**PHENMEDIPHAM:** a contact herbicide used on sugar beet, fodder crops and fruit. Harmful to fish.

**PHENYLMERCURY SALICYLATE:** a seed treatment used in the past on flax, grains, peanuts, peas and soya beans, but withdrawn in the UK in 1972.

**PHORATE:** an organophosphorous insecticide used on vegetables, cotton and maize. Extremely hazardous. In India it has been found that washing fruit and vegetables reduced residues by up to 84%. Dangerous to fish, wild birds and bees. Since 1974 banned for commercial agricultural purposes in Malaysia.

**PHOSALONE:** an organophosphorous insecticide used on fruit, vegetables and cereals. Some evidence of chronic effects in animals. In India it has been found that washing fruit and vegetables reduced residues by between 24% and 73%. Harmful to fish, bees and birds.

**PHOSMET:** an organophosphorous insecticide first registered in the US in 1966 and used on fruit, grapes and potatoes. Evidence of animal carcinogenicity, mutagenicity and reproductive effects. Dangerous to fish and harmful to birds and bees.

**PHOSPHAMIDON:** a very toxic organophosphorous insecticide used on rice, sugar cane and fruit. Some animal evidence of carcinogenicity and mutagenicity. Highly toxic to birds and bees and toxic to wildlife. Not approved for use in the UK.

**PICLORAM:** a translocated herbicide. Some evidence of on-cogenicity in animals. Withdrawn in Sweden in 1984 because of its extreme persistence and environmental impact, and in Finland in 1986 because of insufficient documentation. Data gaps existed in 1980s. Harmful to fish.

**PIRIMICARB:** a carbamate insecticide used on cereals, vegetables and fruit. Some evidence of animal carcinogenicity exists. Harmful to livestock.

**PIRIMIPHOS-METHYL:** an organophosphorous insecticide widely used on crops. Some data on its mutagenicity and reproductive effects in animals does exist. Dangerous to bees and harmful to fish.

**PROCHLORAZ:** a systemic fungicide used on cereals, fruit and vegetables. Dangerous to fish.

**PROPHAM:** a soil-acting carbamate herbicide used on vegetables, fodder crops and sugar beet. Some evidence of animal on-cogenicity. Data gaps existed throughout 1980s including gaps on residues in food. Dangerous to fish.

**PROPICONAZOLE:** a systemic fungicide used on cereals and vines. Harmful to bees and dangerous to fish.

**PRONAMIDE:** potentially oncogenic herbicide used on lettuce in the US since 1972.

**PROPOXUR:** a carbamate insecticide used widely against a range of insect pests. Evidence of mutagenicity exists and of reproductive effects in animals. Harmful to wild birds, animals and fish.

**PYRAZOPHOS:** an organophosphorous fungicide used on cereals, fruit and hops. Some evidence of mutagenicity. Dangerous to bees and harmful to fish and birds.

**PYRINURON:** a rodenticide banned in Sweden in 1980 because of the development of diabetes mellitus in experimental animals exposed to the pesticide.

**QUINTOZENE:** a fungicide which in the past has been contaminated by HCB, an oncogen, and so the US specify maximum HCB levels in the product and control the pesticide's use near water supplies.

**RACEMATE PRODUCTS:** products of dichlorprop and mecoprop banned due to the new registration of one-isomer products in Sweden in 1989.

**RESMETHRIN:** a synthetic pyrethroid insecticide used on food storage, harmful to fish and bees.

**SIMAZINE:** a triazine herbicide first registered in the US in 1957 and used on coffee, fruit, vegetables and cereals. Restricted in Sweden in 1989 – see atrazine. Some evidence of carcinogenicity, mutagenicity and possible reproductive effects in animals. Data gaps including gaps on residues in food existed in the 1980s. Residues have been detected in the USSR on grapes and apples. Do not contaminate water.

**SODIUM CHLORATE:** a herbicide banned in Sweden in 1990 because of its high mobility in soil and insufficient documentation.

**SODIUM FLOUROACETATE and FLOUROACETAMIDE:** a rodenticide used in Western Europe but banned in Philippines.

**SULFALLATE:** a herbicide first registered in the US in 1973. Evidence of animal carcinogenicity and mutagenicity exists. Production discontinued in the US in 1973.

**2,4,5-T:** a phenoxyacetic acid herbicide banned in Sweden in 1977 because of toxic dioxin impurities in commercial products. Also banned in Turkey and Philippines. Harmful to fish.

**TCA:** a herbicide banned in Sweden in 1990 because of its high mobility in soil and insufficient documentation.

**TECNAZENE:** a fungicide and growth regulator used widely on potatoes. Some evidence of animal oncogenicity exists. Residues widely detected in potatoes. Harmful to fish.

**TERBUTRYN:** a triazine herbicide used on cereals, vegetables and sugar cane. Registered in the US since 1969. Potentially oncogenic in animals. Data gaps including gaps on residues existed in the 1980s. May be harmful to fish.

**TETRACHLORVINPHOS:** potentially oncogenic insecticide used on cattle and poultry in the US since 1969.

**TETRAMETHRIN:** a synthetic pyrethroid insecticide. Some evidence of animal carcinogenicity exists. Dangerous to fish and toxic to bees.

**THALLIUM SULPHATE:** withdrawn from the market in Sweden in 1968 because of its high acute toxicity. Banned in the Philippines and in Portugal.

**THIABENDAZOLE:** a systemic fungicide first registered in the US in 1968 and used widely on vegetables, rice, fruit and cereals. Data gaps exist. Some evidence of mutagenicity exists. Apparently banned as a food ingredient in the US in 1990. Harmful to fish.

**THIODICARB:** potentially oncogenic carbamate insecticide used on soya beans and cotton in the US since 1985. Its metabolite, acetamide, is oncogenic at high doses in animals.

**THIOMETON:** an organophosphorous insecticide used on vegetables, cereals and some berries. Highly hazardous. Harmful to bees, fish and birds.

**THIOPHANATE-METHYL:** potentially oncogenic systemic fungicide used on fruit, nuts and vegetables in the US since 1972. Restricted use in Finland because of concern about its toxicity and its metabolite MBC which is mutagenic (see carbendazim).

**THIRAM:** a dithiocarbamate fungicide used on vegetables, fruit and cereals. Some evidence of mutagenicity and reproductive effects in animals at very high doses. Residues found in intact fruit after peeling. Toxic to fish.

**TOXAPHENE:** potentially oncogenic insecticide used on cattle, grain, fruit and vegetables and registered in the US since 1955. Banned in Turkey, Bulgaria and the Philippines; withdrawn in Denmark, New Zealand and Pakistan; not approved for use in the UK. Extremely toxic to fish and harmful to other animals.

**TRIADIMEFON:** a systemic fungicide used on cereals, fruit and vegetables as well as coffee. Harmful to fish.

**TRIADIMENOL:** a systemic fungicide used on fruit and vegetables. Harmful to fish.

**TRIAZOPHOS:** an organophosphorous insecticide used on cereals, fruit and vegetables. Highly hazardous to workers. Dangerous to bees and harmful to fish and birds.

**TRICLOPYR:** a translocated herbicide used on rice, wheat and other crops. Dangerous to fish.

**TRIFLURALIN:** potentially oncogenic herbicide used on soya beans, vegetables and fruit and registered in the US since 1963. Linked to chronic effects and carcinogenicity in animals. May be contaminated by nitrosamines. Harmful to fish.

**UDMH:** an oncogen present in daminozide (see earlier entry) and a breakdown product of that pesticide. Concentrations of the chemical may be increased by cooking fruit treated with daminozide.

**VINCLOZOLIN:** a fungicide first registered in the US in 1981. Mutagenicity has been reported in one laboratory test.

**WAXED PRODUCTS:** a range of food products can be waxed. These include apples in the US, and avocados, cantaloupes, peppers, lemons, peaches, passion fruit, pumpkins, squashes, grapefruits, melons and tomatoes. The FDA in the US approves 6 waxes for 18 types of produce. Waxes may contain shellacs, paraffin, palm oil, synthetic resins and, in some countries, fungicides like benomyl, diphenyl, thiabendazole, ortho-phenylphenol, dicloran and imazalil. According to Ted Parrett in the UK *Food Magazine* in 1990, diphenyl is an animal oncogen and fruit shipped to Germany or Italy must carry the warning label 'with diphenyl – peel unsuitable for consumption'; orthophenylphenol is a potential oncogen; and sodium orthophenylphenate is also linked with mutagenicity and may be used in wax.

**ZINEB:** potentially oncogenic dithiocarbamate fungicide used on fruit, small grains and vegetables in the US since 1955. Restricted use pesticide in Poland for non-edible parts of plants. Toxic to fish at certain levels. (See EBDCs).

**ZIRAM:** an oncogenic dithiocarbamate fungicide used on fruit and vegetables. Evidence of mutagenicity and animal reproductive effects. Harmful to fish.

# PART 4
# Further information

## ABBREVIATIONS

The following abbreviations are widely used in connection with pesticides research, testing and applications and by national and international agro-chemical groups and organisations.

**a.c.** aqueous concentrate.
**ACP** Advisory Committee on Pesticides (UK).
**ADAS** MAFF Agricultural Development and Advisory Service (UK).
**ADI** Acceptable Daily Intake.
**a.i.** active ingredient.
**ANS** autonomic nervous system.
**BAA** British Agro-Chemical Association.
**BASIS** British Agrochemical Supply Industry Scheme.
**BCPC** British Crop Protection Council.
**BHC** benzene hexachloride.
**b.p.** boiling point.
**CAC** (**Codex Alimentarius Commission**) The joint FAO/WHO publication which lists maximum residue limits for pesticides.
**CDA** Controlled Droplet Application.
**Che** cholinesterase.
**CNS** Central Nervous System.
**CPL** Classification, Packaging and Labelling of Dangerous Substances Regulations 1984 (UK).
**2,4-D** 2,4-dichlorophenoxyacetic acid.
**DDT** dichloro diphenyl trichlorethane.
**DDVP** dichlorvos.
**dia** diameter.
**d.p.** dispersible powder.
**EC** effect concentration, specific effect level.

**e.c.** emulsifiable concentrate.

**ED** effect dose, specific effect level.

**EPA** Environmental Protection Agency (US).

**FAO** United Nations Food and Agriculture Organisation.

**FDA** Food and Drugs Administration (US).

**FEPA** Food and Environmental Protection Act (UK).

**FIFRA** Federal Insecticide, Fungicide and Rodenticide Act 1974 (US).

**GIFAP** International Agro-Chemical Industry Federation (Groupe International des Associations Nationales de Fabricants de Produits Agrochimiques).

**GIT** Gastro-Intestinal Tract.

**HASAWA** Health and Safety at Work [etc.] Act of 1974 (UK).

**HCH 1,2,3,4,5,6** hexachlorocyclohexane (or BHC).

**HSC** Health and Safety Commission (a policy body) (UK).

**HSE** Health and Safety Executive (the enforcement agency of HSC) (UK).

**h.v.** high volume.

**IARC** International Agency for Research on Cancer.

**ISO** International Standardisation Organisation.

**LC50** median Lethal Concentration 50 (to kill 50% of test organism).

**LD50** median Lethal Dose 50 (to kill 50% of test organism).

**l.v.** low volume.

**MAC** Maximum Allowable Concentration.

**MAFF** Ministry of Agriculture, Fisheries and Food (UK).

**MCPA** 4-chloro-2-methyl phenoxyacetic acid.

**MDAF** Minimum Dose Always Fatal in 24 hours.

**MDNF** Maximum Dose Never Fatal in 24 hours.

**mg** milligramme.

**ml** millilitre.

**m/m** proportion by mass.

**m.p.** melting point.

**m** micrometre (micron).

**MLD** Minimum Lethal Dose.

**MRL** Maximum Residue Level.

**NEL** No effect level.

**NIOSH** National Institution of Occupational Safety and Health (US).

**NOEL** No Observable Effect Level.

**NRC** National Research Council (US).

**NRDC** Natural Resources Defense Council: an environmental pressure group (US).

**PAN** Pesticides Action Network (an international body).

**PCP** pentachlorophenol.

**ppb** parts per billion.

**ppm** parts per million.

**post-em** post-emergent. A term which describes herbicides applied to weeds after they have emerged.

**ppmv** parts per million by volume.

**pre-em** pre-emergent. A term used to describe herbicides applied to the ground before weeds appear on the surface.

**RPE** Respiratory Protective Equipment.

**s.c.** suspension concentrate.

**s.p.** soluble powder.

**STEL** Short-term Exposure Limit (for a TLV or OEL).

**2,4,5-T** 2,4,5-trichlorophenoxyacetic acid.

**TC** Toxic Concentration.

**TCDD** 2,3,7,8-tetrachlorodibenzo-*p*-dioxin (often called just 'dioxin').

**TD** Toxic Dose (lowest observed).

**ULV** Ultra-Low volume spraying.

**UNEP** United Nations Environmental Programme.

**VLV** Very Low Volume.

**v.m.d.** volume mean diameter of spray droplet.

**v.p.** vapour pressure.

**v.v.** volume per volume.

**WHO** World Health Organisation.

**w.p.** wettable powder.

**w.s.c.** water soluble concentrate.

**w.s.p.** water soluble powder.

**w/v** weight by volume.

**w.w.** weight by weight.

# GLOSSARY

Some common terms relating to pesticides and their adverse health effects. (Based on the glossary in my *Pesticide Users Health and Safety Handbook* – see Booklist).

**absorption** (dermal) the movement of substances through the skin.

**acaricide** a chemical used to kill mites and ticks.

**acetylcholine** a chemical in the body which acts as a neurotransmitter to nerves in the body.

**activator** a chemical added to a pesticide to increase its activity.

**acute effect** toxicological term for the adverse effect produced by a single short exposure to a substance.

**adenoma** a benign tumour.

**ADI** Acceptable Daily Intake. The amount of a chemical which can be consumed daily for the lifetime of an individual with no ill-effects.

**adjuvant** an inactive chemical which, when added to a pesticide, increases the efficiency of that pesticide, e.g. wetting agents, emulsifiers, dispersing agents.

**aetiology** the study of the causes of diseases.

**agro-chemical** general term for chemicals used in agriculture, including insecticides, fungicides, herbicides, acaricides, veterinary pesticides, medicinal feed additives.

**algicide** a chemical which kills algae.

**allergen** a substance that the body regards as foreign or potentially dangerous (and against which it produces an antibody) and which causes an allergy in hypersensitive people.

**Ames test** a rapid biochemical laboratory test to detect mutagenic chemicals.

**amines** compounds of ammonia.

**amine salts** organic derivatives of ammonia (primary salts = amino base; secondary = iminobase salts; tertiary = nitrite salts).

**aphicide** a chemical used to kill aphids.

**aromatic compounds** related to benzene and including toluene, xylene and trimethyl benzene.

**ataxia** shaky movements and unsteady gait due to neurological problems (often an indication of some forms of pesticide poisoning). Organic mercury pesticides and organophosphorous pesticides can cause ataxia.

**attractant** a substance for attracting pests to control or destroy them, e.g. use of a pheromone.

**autonomic nervous system** the part of the nervous system responsible for the control of the bodily functions that are not consciously directed, e.g. the heart beat, sweating, salivation, intestinal activity. Pesticides can disrupt this system, especially organophosphorous insecticides.

**biocide** chemical used to kill bacteria, fungus, etc.

**biological control** regulation of plant and animal populations by natural enemies.

**bipyridilium compounds** a group of herbicides that includes diquat and paraquat.

**bradycardia** slowing of the heart rate to less than 50 beats per minute (a possible symptom of carbamate poisoning).

**carbamate** one of a group of synthetic organic insecticides in the carbamate group which contain carbon, hydrogen and sulfur and are anti-cholinesterase agents (e.g. bendiocarb and carbaryl).

**carcinogen** a cancer-causing substance. Cancer is any malignant tumour.

**carrier** the liquid or solid substances added to a herbicide as a dilutant to aid application and to carry the pesticide to its target.

**chemical name** specific name for an active pesticide ingredient which may vary from country to country.

**cholinergic** activated by acetylcholine.

**cholinesterase (Che)** an enzyme in the body which breaks down the neurotransmitter, acetylcholine, after it has relayed nerve impulses. Some pesticides, especially organophosphorous ones, interfere with this process and so affect the nervous system and prevent proper nerve function.

**chromosomes** the parts of the nucleus of a cell which transmit genetic information.

**chronic exposure** prolonged or repeated exposure to a substance.

**chronic poisoning** poisoning resulting from cumulative damage after exposure to small amounts of a pesticide after long or repeated exposure.

**clastogen** the general class of substances which produce alterations in the cell chromosomes.

**co-carcinogen** a substance that enhances the effects of a carcinogen.

**common name** simple or well-known name of a pesticide.

**contact herbicide** one which causes local damage to plant tissue where contact occurs (same for contact insecticide but damage is to insect).

**controlled droplet application** the method used to try to ensure that pesticides are applied in drops of approximately similar size.

**crop protectant** an additive to a herbicide which reduces the adverse effects on a crop.

**cumulative dose** the effects of increasing amounts of a substance building up in the body.

**defoliant** a pesticide which causes the leaves of plants to fall (phenoxy acetic acid herbicides have been widely used for this purpose).

**dermatitis** inflammation of the skin from any cause.

**desiccant** a pesticide which causes the dehydration of a plant tissue and so causes it to dry out, wither and die (diquat is used as a desiccant).

**dinitro compounds** this group of insecticides contains DNOC and dinoseb.

**dispersing agent** a material or substance that reduces the attraction between like particles.

**dithiocarbamate fungicides** this group of pesticides contain and zineb.

**diuresis** increased production of urine.

**dust** a suspension of particles in the air. Non-toxic dusts are called 'nuisance' dusts but these may present hazards if inhaled in large quantities. Also, so-called nuisance dusts have later proved to be toxic. A wide range of herbicides and insecticides may be applied as granules with a possible dust risk to applicators, e.g. aldicarb.

**dysarthia** speech disorder in which the pronunciation is unclear (possible symptom of organic mercury poisoning).

**dyspnoea** laboured or difficult breathing (a possible symptom of carbamate poisoning).

**endogenous chemical** chemicals produced by or found naturally in the body.

**epidemiology** the study of the frequency of cases of a particular disease related to geographical location.

**epigenetic carcinogens** carcinogens which act by an indirect mechanism and do not affect cell genetic information.

**epistaxis** nose bleed (may be a symptom of inhalation of paraquat/diquat).

**erythema** abnormal flushing of the skin.

**erythrocytes** red blood cells.

**esters** derivatives of acids made by replacing hydrogens with alkyl radicals, e.g. 2,4-D herbicide.

**exogenous chemical** one produced not in the body but derived from outside.

**foaming agent** additive to pesticide which helps to stop spray drift by forming a thick foam in the pesticide.

**formulation** a pesticide prepared in a form suitable for practical use: the technical formulation of a pesticide applied in the field may well vary from the original laboratory preparation of a pesticide.

**fungicides** pesticides used to treat fungus problems in agriculture and within buildings.

**gene** a part of the chromosome.

**genotoxic carcinogens** carcinogens which interfere with the genetic information in the cells.

**genotoxicity** that which is toxic to the gene.

**halogens** inorganic chemicals containing one or more of the following: fluorine, chlorine, bromine, iodine.

**hepatic** relating to the liver.

**herbicide** a chemical used to kill unwanted plants.

**hypopnoea** decrease in breathing rate (a possible symptom of carbamate poisoning).

**immune system** the system in the body which deals with resistance to infection.

**ingested** swallowed, accidentally or deliberately: in a powder or granular form pesticides may be ingested, sometimes on food, on hands and fingers when smoking, or even on chewing gum/tobacco.

**inhaled** breathed in.

**inorganic chemicals** those not containing carbon.

**insecticides** groups of pesticides used to control insects.

**in vitro** experiments in a test tube or other similar laboratory container on living organisms, often micro-organisms.

**in vivo** experiments on the living animal.

**isomer** one of at least two substances in which the molecules contain the same number of atoms but are differently arranged so that each isomer has different properties. e.g. HCH.

**latent period** time between exposure to the cause of a disease (e.g. a toxic pesticide) and the onset of the disease, possibly many years later.

**larvacide** insecticide used to kill insect larvae.

**lipid** any group of organic substances (e.g. fat) that does not dissolve in water. General term for oils, fats, waxes found in living tissue.

**lymphoma** a malignant tumour of the lymph nodes excluding Hodgkin's disease.

**maximum residue limit (MRL)** maximum concentration of a pesticide residue permitted in food on harvest or before consumption.

**metabolism** the process by which chemicals are altered and broken down or built up in the cells of the body tissues, mostly by enzymes.

**micron (n)** one thousandth part of a millimetre.

**miscible** two or more liquids which can be mixed and will stay mixed under normal conditions.

**mist** air-borne suspensions of liquid droplets.

**molluscicide** pesticide used to control slugs and snails.

**mutagen** those substances which induce transmissible changes in the genetic material carried by reproductive cells, both male and female.

**myotonia** abnormally prolonged muscle contractions and stiffness (may be a symptom of phenoxyacetic acid poisoning).

**narcosis** stupor or drowsiness and unconsciousness caused by chemical substances.

**neoplasm** a new growth consisting of abnormal cells: a tumour.

**nephritis** inflammation of the kidney.

**neurological** relating to the study of the structure, functioning and diseases of the nervous system.

**non-selective pesticide** a chemical which is toxic to plants or insects without regard to species.

**oncogen** in this context a substance which may cause either a benign or a malignant tumour.

**organic compound** those which contain carbon atoms.

**organochlorine pesticides** those pesticides containing one or more chlorine atoms (e.g. lindane, chlordane). Sometimes called chlorinated hydrocarbons.

**organophosphorous pesticides** those pesticides containing a phosphorous atom (e.g. malathion, dichlorvos, etc.).

**ovicide** a pesticide which kills insect eggs before they hatch.

**papilloma** a benign tumour.

**paraesthesiae** abnormal tingling sensations, and numbness symptoms of partial damage to peripheral nerves (may be a symptom of methyl bromide poisoning).

**peripheral neuropathy/neuritis** loss of co-ordination in the extremities due to damage to the nervous system.

**pesticide** general term used to cover herbicides, insecticides, fungicides, acaricides, etc.

**phenoxyacetic acid herbicides** herbicides containing hydroxyl and acid substitutes (e.g. 2,4-D and 2,4,5-T).

**pheromones** chemicals secreted by insects which attract other insects (e.g. aggregating pheromones and sex pheromones).

**phytotoxic** toxic to plants, normally the higher or green plants.

**plant regulator** chemical used to restrain growth of bushes, cereals, grasses.

**polyneuropathy** disease involving all the peripheral nerves.

**post-emergent** refers to the application of a herbicide after a crop has emerged above the soil.

**potentiation** increase of power of a pesticide.

**pre-emergent** refers to the application of a chemical, usually a herbicide, on a crop after sowing of seed but before the crop has emerged.

**promoter** a chemical which enhances the development of a cancer after cells have been exposed to carcinogens without becoming cancerous. The promoters themselves may not be carcinogens.

**reproductive toxicity effects** includes not only teratogenicity, mutagenicity and carcinogenicity but also effects on fertility, libido, menstruation, etc.

**residual pesticide** one which remains active in the soil for a period of time.

**rodenticide** pesticide used to kill rats, mice and other rodents.

**safener** a chemical which reduces the adverse effects of a herbicide on a crop and hence enhances selectivity (same as 'crop protectant').

**sarcoma** any cancer of connective tissue.

**sensitisation** abnormal sensitivity to a chemical: once sensitised, a person may react to very low levels of the sensitising chemical thereafter.

**solvent** a liquid that is capable of dissolving other substances.

**spray drift**  drift of pesticide droplets away from the target area.

**stomatitis**  inflammation of the mucous lining of the mouth (a sign of arsenical poisoning).

**surfactant**  a substance which, when added to a pesticide, reduces tension on plants and increases the spreading, wetting and emulsifying properties of the pesticide application.

**synapse**  gap across which nerve impulses pass from one neurone to the next at the end of a nerve fibre.

**synergism**  the process whereby one chemical interacts with another to produce increased activity.

**synthetic pyrethroids**  this group of insecticides are similar in structure to the naturally occurring pyrethroids and contain cypermethrin, deltamethrin, etc.

**systemic effect**  one relating to or affecting the body as a whole, rather than individual parts and organs.

**systemic pesticide**  one which enters a plant either by its roots or leaves and is translocated within it.

**tachycardia**  an increase of the heart rate above normal (a possible symptom of pentachlorophenol poisoning).

**tank mix**  two or more pesticides or other chemicals mixed in a spray tank prior to application.

**tenesmus**  sensation of the desire to defecate which is continuous or recurs frequently (a possible symptom of organophosphorous poisoning).

**teratogen**  any substance which causes malformations in the foetus.

**trade name**  manufacturer's commercial name for a pesticide.

**translocated pesticide**  one where the pesticide moves within the plant.

**triazine herbicides**  this group contains simazine, atrazine, etc.

**vapour**  a gas often produced by the evaporation of a volatile liquid such as propionic acid.

**vapour drift**  movement of a pesticide in the form of vapour away from the target area. 2,4-D in ester form is a volatile pesticide likely to drift.

**vector**  a carrier, usually an insect carrying either human or plant diseases.

**volatility**  substances, usually liquids, which evaporate easily to form a vapour or a gas.

**wettable powder**  a pesticide powder formulation which is dispersed in water.

# BOOKLIST

The most up-to-date and comprehensive guides to pesticide chemistry and properties are the Pesticide Manual (British Crop Protection Council, 1990), and the Royal Society of Chemistry's loose-leafed *Agro-Chemical Handbook*. The contents of both these books are now available through computerised data bases.

Various environmental and worker groups have produced useful and lucid guides to hazardous pesticides, pesticides poisoning and pollution. Booklets by the National Wildlife Federation in Washington and Friends of the Earth in Britain (*Pesticides Incidents Reports* in the 1980s) are probably the most useful.

The British publications on the medical and environmental problems of pesticides are very sparse. The one government guide – produced by the DHSS in 1983 – was prepared not solely by independent specialists in the field but in conjunction with the British Agro-chemicals Association Ltd. (the manufacturers' trade group).

Guides to veterinary pesticides and animal feed additives which fall within the agro-chemical definition tend to have less information available in them on human and environmental problems than those on pesticides used for crop treatments.

Three British guides cover nomenclature and technical rather than health and safety usage:

1. *Guide to Veterinary Pesticides* (MAFF, 2nd ed., 1984).
2. *Compendium of Data Sheets for Veterinary Products,* 1989-90, NOAH (Data Pharm Publications, London, 1989).
3. *Handbook of Medicinal Feed Additives* (HMG Publications, Bakewell, 1983).

The latter two guides tend to be updated at frequent intervals, if not annually, but only the NOAH publication contains human health and safety information.

Abelson, P.H., 'Testing for Carcinogens in Rodents', *Science* 249; 1357, 21 September 1990.

Andresson, A., T. Bergh, et al, *Pesticides Residues in Fruit and Vegetables in Sweden, 1989* (Uppsala, 1990), SV Report 4.

Barlow, S. and E. Sullivan *Reproductive Hazards of Industrial Chemicals* (Academic Press, London, 1982).

Berg, G.L., *Farm Chemicals Handbook 1985* (Meister Co., Willoughby, Ohio, 1985.

Boardman, R., *Pesticides in World Agriculture* (Macmillan, Basingstoke, 1986).

Body, R., *Agriculture: the Triumph and the Shame* (Temple Smith, London, 1982).

British Agro-Chemical Association, *Directory of Garden Chemicals*, 1988/9 edition (BAA, Peterborough, 1989).

British government publications: Select Committee on Agriculture, *The Effects of Pesticides on Human Health, Vol. 1, Report and Proceedings* (HMSO, London, 1987). Advisory Committee on Pesticides, *Annual Reports 1985, 1986, 1987, 1988* (HMSO, London, 1986 to 1990).

Bull, D., *A Growing Problem: Pesticides and the Third World Poor* (Oxfam, Oxford, 1982).

Bust, R., *Food Chemical Sensitivity,* (Prism, Bridport, 1986).

Carson, R., *Silent Spring* (Penguin Books, Harmondsworth, 1966).

Conning, D.M. and A.B.G. Lansdown, *Toxic Hazards in Food* (Croom Helm, London, 1983).

Cook, J. and C. Kaufman, *Portrait of a Poison: the 2,4,5-T Story* (Pluto Press, London, 1982).

Debach, Paul, *Biological Control of Natural Enemies* (Cambridge University Press, London, 1974).

DHSS, *Pesticide Poisoning: Notes for the Guidance of Medical Practioners* (HMSO, London, 1983).

Doyal, L. et al., *Cancer in Britain* (Pluto Press, London, 1983).

Dreisbach, R.H., *A Handbook of Poisoning*, 11th edn. (Lange Medical Publications, Los Altos, California, 1983).

Dudley, N, *How Does Your Garden Grow: A Guide to the Effects of Garden Chemicals* (Soil Association, Bristol, 1986).

Duffus, J.H., *Environmental Toxicology* (Edward Arnold, London, 1980).

Ecobichon, D.J. and R.M. Joy, *Pesticides and Neurological Diseases* (CRC Press, Boca Raton, Florida, 1982).

Elkington, J., *The Poisoned Womb: Human Reproduction in a Poisoned World* (Viking, Harmondsworth, 1985).

Environmental Data Services (ENDS), *Report No. 138* (ENDS, London, 1986).

Epstein, S., *The Politics of Cancer* (Sierra Club Books, San Francisco, 1978).

Erlichman, J., *Gluttons for Punishment* (Penguin, Harmondsworth, 1986).

Fairchild, E.J. (ed.), *Agricultural Chemicals and Pesticides: A Handbook of Toxic Effects, A NIOSH Sub-File* (Castle House Publications, Guildford, 1978).

Fan, A.M. and R.J. Jackson, 'Pesticides and Food Safety', *Regulatory Toxicology and Pharmacology*, 9 (1989).

Fletcher, A., *Reproductive Hazards of Work* (Equal Opportunities Commission, Manchester, 1985).

FAO/WHO, *Codex Maximum Limits for Pesticide Residues*, 2nd edn. (Rome, 1986, 1988). Vol XIII and Supplement 1 of the CAC.

Frankel, M., *Chemical Risk* (Pluto, London, 1982).

Frankel, M., *A Word of Warning: The Quality of Chemical Suppliers Health and Safety Information* (Social Audit, London, 1981).

George, S., *How the Other Half Dies* (Penguin Books, Harmondsworth, 1976).

Gibson, G.G. and R. Walker, *Food Toxicology – Real or Imaginary Problems?* (Taylor and Francis, London, 1985).

Gillespie, B., D. Eva and R. Johnston, 'Carcinogenic Risk Assessment in the United States and Great Britain: the Case of Aldrin/Dieldrin', *Social Studies of Science*, 9 (1977).

Gosselin, R.E., R.P. Smith and H.C. Hodge, *Clinical Toxicology of Commercial Products*, 5th edn. (Williams and Wilkins, Baltimore/London, 1984).

Goulding, R., 'Poisoning on the Farm', *Journal of the Society of Occupational Medicine*, 33 (1983).

*Great Britain: The Pesticides (Maximum Residue Limits in Food) Regulations 1988* (HMSO, London, 1988).

Green, M.B., G.S. Hartley and T.F. West, *Chemicals for Crop Protection and Pest Control*, 2nd rev. edn. (Pergamon Press, Oxford, 1979).

Greenhalgh, R. and T. Roberts, *Pesticide Science and Technology* (Blackwell, Oxford, 1987).

Gunn, D.L. and G.R. Stevens, *Pesticides and Human Welfare* (Oxford University Press, Oxford, 1976).

Guthrie, F. and J.J. Perry, eds., *Introduction to Environmental Toxicology* (Elsevier, New York, 1980). Especially pp. 200-312.

Hall, R.H., *A New Approach to Pest Control in Canada* (Ottawa, 1981). Canadian Environmental Advisory Council Report 10.

Hallenbeck, W.H. and K.M. Cunningham-Burns, *Pesticides and Human Health* (Springer Verlag, New York, 1985).

Hassall, K.A., *The Chemistry of Pesticides* (Macmillan, London, 1982).

Hay, A., *The Chemical Scythe: Lessons of 2,4,5-T and Dioxin* (Plenum Press, New York, 1982).

Hayes, W.J., *Pesticides Studied in Man* (Williams and Wilkins, Baltimore and London, 1982).

Health and Safety Commission, *Methods for the Determination of Toxicity: Approved Code of Practice* (HMSO, London, 1982).

Health and Safety Commission, *Methods for the Determination of Ecotoxicity: Approved Code of Practice* (HMSO, London, 1982).

Health and Safety Executive, *Notification of New Substances Regulations: A Guide* (HMSO, London, 1982).

International Agency for Research on Cancer, *Some Halogenated Hydrocarbons and Pesticide Exposure* (IARC, Lyon, 1986), IARC Monograph 41.

ILO, *Occupational Exposure Limits*, 2nd rev. edn. (ILO, Geneva, 1980).

ILO, *Safe Use of Pesticides* (ILO, Geneva, 1977).

IOCU, *The Pesticides Handbook* (IOCU, Penang, 1984).

Isa, A.L., 'Pesticides Regulations in Egypt to Avoid Hazards to the Environment and Human Health', *Journal of Environmental Science and Health,* B15(6), (1980).

Jeyaratnam, J., 'Agriculture in the Third World', in J.C. McDonald, ed., *Recent Advances in Occupational Health: Number 1* (Churchill Livingstone, Edinburgh 1981).

Jeyaratnam, J., R.S. de Alwis Seneviratne and J.F. Copplestone, 'Survey of Pesticide Poisoning in Sri Lanka', *Bulletin of WHO,* 60, 4 (1982).

Jeyaratnam, I., 'Health Problems of Pesticide Usage in the Third World', *British Journal of Industrial Medicine* 42 (1985).

Lappe, F.M. and J. Collins, *Food First* (Abacus, London, 1982).

Lashford, S., *The Residue Report* (Thorsons, Wellingborough, 1988).

Levnedsmiddelstyrelsen, *Pesticides in Danish Food* (Copenhagen, 1987).

Lodeman, E.G., *The Spraying of Plants* (Macmillan, New York/London, 1986).

Loevinsohn, M.E., 'Insecticide Use and Increased Mortality in Rural Central Luzon, Philippines' *Lancet,* 13 June 1987.

London Food Commission, *Food Adulteration and How to Beat it* (Unwin Paperbacks, London, 1988).

MAFF, Report of the Working Party on Pesticide Residues: 1985-1988 (HMSO,London, 1989).

MAFF, *A Guide to Veterinary Products,* 2nd edn. (HMSO, London, 1984). MAFF Reference Book 245.

MAFF, *Pesticides 1990* (HMSO, London, 1990).

MAFF, Report of the Working Party on Pesticide Residues: 1988-1989 (HMSO, London, 1990).

Matsumura, F., *Toxicology of Pesticides* (Plenum Press, New York, 1975).

Matsumura, F., G.M. Boush and T. Misato, ed., *Environmental Toxicology of Pesticides* (Academic Press, New York, 1972).

Matthews, G.A., *Pesticide Application Methods* (Longman, London, 1979).

Mellanby, K., *Pesticides and Pollution* (Collins, London, 1967).

Morgan, D.P., *Recognition and Management of Pesticide Poisoning*, 3rd edn. (EPA, Washington, 1982).

Mott, L. and K. Snyder, *Pesticide Alert: A Guide to Pesticides in Fruit and Vegetables* (Sierra Club Books, San Francisco, 1987).

Napompeth, B., *Thailand: National Profile on Pest Management and Related Problems* (National Research Council, Bangkok, 1981).

National Research Council, *Regulating Pesticides in Food* (National Academy Press, Washington, 1987).

National Wildlife Federation, *34 Pesticides: Is Safe Use Possible* (NWF, Washington, 1984).

New South Wales Health Commission, *Poisoning by Pesticides* (Sydney, 1979).

North Carolina State University, *North Carolina Agricultural Chemicals Manual* (College of Agriculture, Raleigh, North Carolina, 1988).

National Institute of Occupational Safety and Health, *Pocket Guide to Chemical Hazards* (DHEW, Washington, 1985).

Oudejans, J.H., *Agro-Pesticides: their Management and Application* (UN, ESCAP, Bangkok, 1982).

Parker, D.V. and R. Truhaut, 'Evaluation of Risks from Pesticide Residues in Food', in Gibson and Walker, *op. cit.*

Parratt, T., *Name Your Poison: A Guide to Additives in Drinks* (Robert Hale, London, 1990).

Pascoe, D., *Toxicology* (Edward Arnold, London, 1983).

Patton, J., *Additives, Adulterants and Contaminants in Beer* (Patton Publications, Barnstaple, 1989).

Perera, F., 'Quantitative Risk Assessment and Cost-Benefit Analysis for Carcinogens: A Critique', *Journal of Public Health Policy* 6: (1987).

Perkins, J.H., *Insects, Experts and the Insecticide Crisis: the Quest for New Pest Management Strategies* (Plenum Press, New York, 1982).

Pimentel, D, and J. Perkins, *Pest Control: Cultural and Environmental Aspects* (Westview Press, Boulder, Calorado, 1980).

Pimentel, D. et al., 'Pesticides: Environmental and Social Costs', in D. Pimentel and J.H. Perkins, *op. cit.*

Pimentel, D., G. Berari and S. Fast, 'Energy Efficiency and Farming Systems: Organic and Conventional Agriculture', *Agriculture, Ecosystems and the Environment*, 9 (1983).

Ragsdale, N.N. and R.E. Menzer, *Carcinogenicity and Pesticides: Principles, Issues and Relationships* (American Chemical Society, Washington, 1989).

Ritchie M. 'GATT, Agriculture and the Environment', *The Ecologist:* 20, 6 (1990).

Royal Commission on Environmental Pollution, *Seventh Report: Agriculture and Pollution* (HMSO, London, 1979).

Royal Society, *Long-term Toxic Effects: A Study Group Report* (Royal Society, London, 1978).

Royal Society of Chemistry, *The Agro-Chemical Handbook* (Royal Society of Chemistry, Nottingham, 1989). And updates.

Salisbury, E., *Weeds and Aliens* (Collins, London, 1961).

Sax, N.I., *Dangerous Properties of Industrial Materials,* 7th edn. (Van Nostrand Reinhold Company, New York, 1989).

Sitting, M., ed., *Pesticide Manufacturing and Toxic Materials Control Encyclopaedia* (Noyes Data Corporation, Park Ridge, New Jersey, 1980).

Snell, P. and K. Nicol, *Pesticides and Residues: the Case for Real Control* (London Food Commission, London, 1986).

Soil Association, *Pall of Poison: the Spray Drift Problem* (Soil Association, Stowmarket, 1984).

Swedish National Food Administration, *Foreign Substances in Food 1989* (NFA, Uppsala, 1989).

Swezey, S.L., R.G. Daxl and D.L. Murray, *Getting off the Pesticides Treadmill in the Developing World: Nicaragua's Revolution in Pesticides Policy* (National University of Nicaragua, Leon, 1984). Mimeo.

UNEP, *Consolidated List of Products whose Consumption and/or Sale have been Banned, Withdrawn, Severely Restricted or Not Approved by Governments,* 2nd issue (UN, New York, 1987).

USA EPA, *Pesticides Fact Handbook* (Noyes Data Corporation, Park Ridge, New Jersey, 1988).

USA EPA, Office of Drinking Water, *Drinking Water Advisory: Pesticides* (Lewis Publishers, Chelsea, Michigan, 1989).

USA FDA, *Residues in Food: 1988* (FDA, Washington, 1989).

Vainio, H., K. Hemminki and J. Wilbourn, 'Data on the Carcinogenicity of Chemicals in the IARC Monograph Program', *Carcinogenesis,* 6 (1985).

Van den Bosch, R., *The Pesticide Conspiracy* (Prism Press, Dorchester, 1980).

Van den Bosch, R. and P.S. Messenger, *Biological Control* (Intertext Books, Leighton Buzzard, 1973).

Watterson, A.E., 'More Effective Control of Pesticides', *Occupational Health,* 34, 9 (1982).

Watterson, A.E., 'Pesticide Health and Safety Policy in the UK: a Flawed and Limited Approach', *Journal of Public Health Policy,* 9 (1990).

Watterson, A.E., *Pesticide Users' Health and Safety Handbook: an International Guide* (Gower Technical, Aldershot, 1988).

Watterson, A.E., 'UK Pesticide Health and Safety Regulatory Policy', *British Journal of Public Health Medicine,* 12 (1990).

Weinstein, S., *Fruits of Your Labor: A Guide to Pesticides Hazards for California Field Workers* (University of California, Berkeley, 1984).

Weir, D. and M. Schapiro, *Circle of Poison: Pesticides and People in a Hungry World* (IFDP, San Francisco, 1981).

WHO/IPCS, *Principles for the Toxicological Assessment of Pesticide Residues in Food* (WHO, Geneva, 1990). *EH Criteria Document 104.*

WHO, *Toxicology of Pesticides: Health Aspects of Chemical Safety Interim Document No. 9* (WHO, Regional Office for Europe, Copenhagen, 1982).

WHO, *WHO Recommended Classification of Pesticides by Hazard: 1986-1987* (WHO, Geneva, 1987).

# USEFUL ORGANIZATIONS TO CONTACT FOR FURTHER INFORMATION

## (1) Official sources of information and advice

### United Kingdom

**Ministry of Agriculture, Fisheries and Food (MAFF),** Ergon House, Horseferry Road, London (Tel 071-270 8080).

**Pesticide Registration Department,** Hatching Green, Harpenden, Herts AL5 2BD (Tel 058 271 5241). Involved in pesticide residue work for MAFF.

### United States

**Environmental Protection Agency (EPA),** 401 M Street SW, Washington DC 20460.

**Food and Drugs Administration (FDA),** Department of Health and Human Services, 5600 Fishers Lane, Rockville, MD 20857.

# (2) Other sources of information and advice

## United Kingdom

**Royal Society of Chemistry,** Thomas Graham House, Science Park, Milton Road, Cambridge CB4 4WF. Produces numerous useful books and journals on agro-chemicals.

## International

**United Nations Food and Agriculture Organisation (FAO),** Via delle Terme di Caracalla, 1-00100 Rome, Italy.

## UN inter-agency bodies

**Codex Committee on Pesticide Residues,** Joint FAO/WHO Food Standards Programme, FAO, (address as above) is the main source of international information on pesticide maximum residue limits and acceptable daily intakes.

**JMPR** (Joint Meeting of FAO Panel of Experts on Pesticide Residues), (address as for FAO).

# (3) Non-governmental agencies

## United Kingdom

**British Organic Farmers and Growers,** 86/88 Colston Street, Bristol BS1 5BB (Tel 0272-299666).

**Food Commission,** 88 Old Street, London EC1V 9AR (Tel 071-250 1021). Produces the *Food Magazine* which covers residues and other subjects relating to pesticides.

**Soil Association,** 86/88 Colston Street, Bristol BS1 5BB (Tel 0272-290661).

**Pesticides Trust,** c/o WUS, 20 Compton Terrace, London N1 (Tel 071-354 3860).

**Parents for Safe Food,** Britannia House, 1-11 Glenthorne Road, London W6 0LF (Tel 01-748 9898).

**Consumers Association,** 2 Marylebone Road, London NW1 4DX (Tel 071-486 5544). Produces *Which?* magazine with useful research on pesticides and food additives.

**Friends of the Earth,** 26-28 Underwood Street, London N1 7JQ (Tel 071-490 1555).

**CAMRA (Campaign for Real Ale),** Information Section, 34 Alma Road, St Albans, Herts AL1 3BW (Tel 0727-86701). Provides information about additives and contaminants in beer.

**Vegetarian Society: Research Section,** Parkdale, Dunham Road, Altrincham, Cheshire WA14 4QG (Tel 061-928 0793). A good source of information on pesticide residues in food.

## United States

**Natural Resources Defense Council (NRDC),** 90 New Montgomery Street, San Francisco, California 94105, USA (Tel (415) 777-0220). Has produced some of the most extensive guides and criticisms on the hazards of pesticide residues in food.

**National Coalition Against Misuse of Pesticides (NCAMP),** 530 Seventh Street SE, Washington DC 2003, USA (Tel (202) 543-5450).

**North West Coalition Against Pesticides (NCAP),** PO Box 1393, Eugene, Oregon, 97440, USA (Tel (503) 344-5044). Produces the *Journal of Pesticide Reform* which is packed with useful articles on pesticides.

## International

**Pesticides Action Network (PAN).** In Europe: Marianne Wenning c/o IDCDA, Bollandistenstraat 22, B-1040 Brussels, Belgium. In the US: Monica Moore, Pesticides Education and Action Project, PO Box 610, San Francisco CA 94101 (Tel (415) 771-7327).

## (4) Industry sources of information and advice

**British Agro-chemical Association,** 4 Lincoln Court, Lincoln Road, Peterborough PE1 2RP (Tel 0733-49255).

**GIFAP** (International Group of National Associations of Agro-chemical Manufacturers), Avenue Albert Lancaster 79A, B-1180 Brussels, Belgium.

# COMMON TRADE NAMES FOR PESTICIDE ACTIVE INGREDIENTS USED BY GARDENERS AND GROWERS

The following list gives widely used trade names to assist UK gardeners and growers. Agro-chemical companies produce many pesticides. Only where the company name is part of the trade name will it be included in the list below. Manufacturers do alter their formulations and always state the principal active ingredients on their labels. You should therefore check the labels on your pesticides to find out which pesticide active ingredients are present now. You should also read the safety precautions carefully before use and storage. Trade names may vary from country to country.

**Trade name** followed by **pesticide active ingredient**

Ambush 1A: PERMETHRIN
Ambush C: CYPERMETHRIN
Atlat Herbon Thuricide: BACILLUS THURINGIENSIS
Avenge H: DIFENZOQUAT METHYL SULPHATE
Basagran: BENTAZONE
Benlate: BENOMYL
Bio Crop Saver: PERMETHRIN, MALATHION
Bio Long Last: DIMETHOATE, PERMETHRIN
Bio Multiveg: PERMETHRIN, CARBENDAZIM, SULPHUR AND OTHERS
Bio Sprayday: PERMETHRIN, PIPERONYL BUTOXIDE
Blackfly and Greenfly Killer: PYRETHRUM, RESMETHRIN
Boots Caterpillar and Whitefly Killer: PERMETHRIN
Boots Garden Fungicide: CARBENDAZIM
Boots Garden Insect Powder: CARBARYL, ROTENONE
Boots Greenfly and Blackfly Killer: DIMETHOATE
Boots Kill-a-Bug: PERMETHRIN, BIOALLETHRIN
Bordeaux Mixture: COPPER SULPHATE
Bug Gun for Fruit and Vegetables: NATURAL PYRETHRUM
Calomel Dust: MERCUROUS CHLORIDE
Casoron H: DICHLOBENIL
Cheshunt Compound: COPPER SULPHATE, AMMONIUM CARBONATE
Clean Up: TAR ACIDS
Couch and Grass Killer: DALAPON
Derris Dust: ROTENONE
Dithane 945: MANCOZEB
Fumite General Purpose Greenhouse Insecticide/Fungicide Smokes:
   PIRIMIPHOS-METHYL
Fumite Tecnalin Greenhouse Insecticide/Fungicide Smokes: LINDANE,
   TECNAZENE
Fumite Whitefly Greenhouse Insecticide Smokes: PERMETHRIN
Gamma-col: LINDANE
Gesaprim: ATRAZINE

Gramoxone H: PARAQUAT DICHLORIDE
Greenhouse and Garden Insect Killer: PYRETHRUM, RESMETHRIN
Herbon Garden Herbicide: PROPHAM, CHLORPROPHAM, DIURON
Hexyl: GAMMA-HCH, ROTENONE, THIRAM
Hostathion: TRIAZOPHOS
ICI Club Root Control: MERCUROUS CHLORIDE
Keriroot: 1-NAPHTHYLACETIC ACID
Kerispray: PIRIMIPHOS-METHYL
Liquid Club Root Control: THIOPHANATE-METHYL
Liquid Derris: ROTENONE
Maldison: MALATHION
Medo: CRESYLIC ACID
Metasystox: DEMETON-S-METHYL
Murphy Combined Seed Dressing: CAPTAN, HCH
Murphy Greenhouse Aerosol: MALATHION
Murphy Mortegg: TAR OILS
Murphy Pest and Disease Smoke: GAMMA-HCH, TECNAZENE
Murphy Systemic Insecticide: DIMETHOATE
Murphy Tumblebite: PROPICONAZOLE
Murphy Tumblebug: PERMETHRIN, HEPTENOPHOS
Nimrod T: BUPIRIMATE, TRIFORINE
Phosdrin: MEVINPHOS
Picket: PERMETHRIN
Pounce: PERMETHRIN
Primatol S: SIMAZINE
Py Garden Insecticide: PYRETHRUM, PIPERONYL BUTOXIDE
Py Powder: PYRETHRUM, PIPERONYL BUTOXIDE
Rapid Aerosol: PIRIMICARB
Rapid Greenfly Killer: PIRIMICARB
Reglone H: DIQUAT DIBROMIDE
Root Guard: DIAZINON
Rooting Powder: CAPTAN, 1-NAPHTHYLACETIC ACID
Roundup: GLYPHOSATE
Rovral F: IPRODIONE
Sevin: CARBARYL
Spring Spray: BROMOPHOS
Slug Guard: METHIOCARB
Slug Pellets (Boots, Fisons, ICI, Murphy Slugit): METALDEHYDE
Strike: CAPTAN, 1-NAPHTHYLACETIC ACID
Supercarb: CARBENDAZIM
Sybol: PIRIMIPHOS-METHYL
Sydane: CHLORDANE
System Fungicide Liquid: THIOPHANATE-METHYL

Systox: DEMETON
Talon 1: CHLORPYRIFOS
Temik: ALDICARB
Tordon 22K: PICLORAM
Tumbleweed: GLYPHOSATE
Verdone 2: MECOPROP, 2,4-D
Weed Gun: 2,4-D, DICAMBA
Weed Out Couchgrass Killer: ALLOXYDIM SODIUM
Weedazol: AMINOTRIAZOLE
Weedex: SIMAZINE
Weedol: PARAQUAT, DIQUAT

# PROGRAMME OF ACTION FOR IMPROVING THE CONTROL OF PESTICIDES AND POTENTIAL RESIDUES IN FOOD

## International

● No pesticide should be used in an international context unless methods for the identification and measurement of their residues, metabolites and degradation products are readily available and can be generally adopted.

● No pesticides should be exported from one country to another without the prior informed consent of the importing country.

● No pesticides banned in one country for reasons of occupational and environmental health should be marketed in other countries where similar hazards would prevail.

● No pesticides should be produced or exported if there is international evidence of probable or possible human carcinogenicity or mutagenicity or teratogenicity or reproductive effects.

● All neurotoxic pesticides should be reviewed.

## National governments

● Pesticides should be used only as part of a properly planned and monitored integrated pest management system. (Sweden, Netherlands and Denmark have already committed themselves to reducing the use of pesticides in agriculture by between 25% and 50% into the 1990s.)

● Proper funding should be established to support long-term research into organic farming.

● All foodstuffs should be labelled with details of pre- and post-harvest chemical treatments. Labels to be based on a coding system similar to that for food additives.

● Testing of residues in foods, both home-grown and imported, should be extensive in terms of samples taken and pesticide residues monitored for, along the lines of the Swedish and US systems.

● Lowest published international MRLs should be adopted if lower than CAC MRLs or existing national standards.

● Full testing of every pesticide to meet the highest international standards of pesticide registration and approval. All data on human and environmental toxicity should be disclosed for public scrutiny.

● Public analysts and government residue chemists should be so funded and staffed to ensure that a full and effective residue monitoring programme can be implemented in line with best international practice.

● Government enforcement of pesticide residue controls should be in ministries or departments independent of agricultural production tasks.

● Enforcement agencies should provide proper staffing and funding to ensure that good agricultural practice is observed by growers and that pesticide application rates and harvest intervals are carefully observed. This will be a double check, with residue monitoring, to keep residues below recommended MRLs and ADIs.

● No pesticides should be approved unless there is evidence of their efficiency.

● No new pesticide to be introduced unless it replaces an existing pesticide.

● All genetically engineered pest controls to be subject to a scrutiny similar to that outlined for pesticides.

● All old pesticides not reviewed by 1995 must have approval revoked.

● No pesticide should be approved or have approval continued if identification, monitoring and measurement of residues and metabolites is not routinely possible by analysts.

● All pesticide approval policies must contain both qualitative and quantitative assessment methods and be geared to the best precautionary policy based on the balance of probabilities approach to the scientific evidence.

## Retail trade

Retailers should:

● Label pre-harvest chemical treatments used on any produce they purchase.
● Label post-harvest chemical treatments of foods sold.

In the US in 1989, 2,000 supermarkets agreed to begin phasing out the use of carcinogenic pesticides on fresh fruit and vegetables. Although the stores were not the biggest, nevertheless they had an annual turnover of over $10 billion a year.

A number of supermarkets in the US and Western Europe have adopted pesticide control policies which require suppliers and growers to monitor residues, to use only certain types of approved pesticides on food crops and not to use others, and to observe application rates and harvest intervals. However, as the details of the residue testing are generally not made available and as information on the pesticide control protocols and 'quality assurance' visits to growers are usually not open to public scrutiny, it is difficult to tell exactly how effective such systems are.

Supermarkets should:

● Request suppliers to disclose information on all pesticides used to grow their produce.
● Encourage suppliers to phase out all known or probable carcinogens and mutagens used on fruit and vegetables.
● Not sell any fruit or vegetables treated with neurotoxic pesticides unless a 'no detectable residue standard' is met.
● Avoid pesticides which cannot be detected using practical analytical laboratory methods.
● Call on governments to remove all pesticides from the marketplace which lack a practical detection method.
(Source for the above: USA Consumer Pesticide Project 1990).
● Publish a pesticide use, reduction and control policy.
● Publish or make available details of their pesticide monitoring and surveillance policies and practices with details of the number of residue tests they carry out each year, on which produce and for which chemicals.

## Consumers

Consumers should:

● Call for full pesticide audits on those pesticides used on domestic or imported foodstuffs to be made available by growers, suppliers, retailers and government. A registry system could collect such audits.

● Demand access to the audits from growers, retailers and governments (for information on audits see pp 29-33).
● Demand the labelling, along the German lines, of all pesticides used on the food sold in shops including pre-harvest and post-harvest treatments and storage and processing. Such pesticides could be labelled with code numbers along the lines of 'E for additives' codes.
● Call for the wider use of IPM and organic farming methods both nationally and through retailers who purchase foods from abroad.


# INTERNATIONAL CONTROLS

The levels of pesticide residues or their metabolites are measured, for regulatory purposes, by MRLs (maximum residue levels) which relate to the maximum levels of pesticide residues which are acceptable in the food. Countries interpret the significance of these levels and their breach in different ways.

In the UK it is stressed that breaches of MRLs do not indicate the safety or otherwise of food because the MRLs themselves are guides to the control of pesticides residues in food and indicators of good agricultural practice. They are not viewed as clear lines between healthy and dangerous food. In Sweden, government agencies can prescribe conditions for or prohibit the offering for sale or other handling of food which contains pesticides which exceed the MRLs.

Most countries tend to boast about the strength of their food controls. The UK is no exception. However, the table below shows that UK MRL controls are, on occasions, twice as weak as those used in Sweden and Germany and not uncommonly five times as weak for a range of pesticides and foodstuffs. This may not be a concern for scientists and government ministers: it is undoubtedly a cause of concern for consumers who can see in the UK that the precautionary approach to pesticides does not always exist and that UK standards are far behind some of their European counterparts on pesticide MRLs.

The UK has only some 60 MRLs set down in the 1988 Pesticide MRL regulations with a few additional controls added in the last two years. It is argued that other UK standards are based on those of the WHO/FAO CAC Codex although without the legal force of the regulations of 1988. However, a close examination of this code reveals that CAC MRLs are themselves far from the best international standards available. One study has recently revealed that the United States Environmental Protection Agency and the Food and Drugs Agency have pesticide residue control standards on many foods which are between 2½ and 50 times tighter than those set down by the CAC MRLs (Ritchie 1990 p216). For instance the US EPA pesticide residue limit on permethrin in apples is forty times tougher than the CAC MRL and the FDA limit on DDT in bananas is fifty times tougher than that of the CAC MRL.

These differences in residue standards raise difficult economic and political as well as scientific problems for the world. They should not be used as a means to damage the trade in food from developing countries to developed countries: the former having weaker standards than the latter. Rather, the approach should be to raise the food safety standards for all countries to the higher levels and for agro-chemical companies and governments to work on producing the lowest possible pesticide levels across the globe.

**Maximum residue levels: Comparison of international standards**
**All levels cited in mg/m³**

| Pesticide | Produce | UK | Sweden | Germany |
|---|---|---|---|---|
| Amitrole | apples | 0.05 | N/A | |
| Azinphos-methyl | citrus | 2 | 1 | |
| Carbaryl | lettuce | 10 | | 3 |
| Carbendazim | wheat | 0.5 | 0.1 | |
| Diazinon | tomatoes | 0.5 | 0.3 | |
| Dichlorvos | tomatoes | 0.5 | 0.1 | 0.1 |
| EBDCs | apples | 3 | 1 | |
| Fenitrothion | wheat | 10 | 1 | |
| Malathion | wheat | 8 | 2 | 3 |
| Mevinphos | potatoes | 0.1 | 0.02 | |
| Phosalone | apples | 5 | 1 | |
| | potatoes | 0.1 | 0.05 | |
| Tecnazene | potatoes | 1 | 0.5 | 0.05 |
| Thiabendazole | potatoes | 5 | 0.5 | |

CW00486312

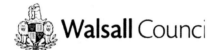

## Walsall Council

This item is due for return on or before

3 000 001 981 21

"In this fast paced and ever changing world our money is held up to the light and marked to check its validity. We are asked almost everywhere for proof of id, to see if we are who we say we are. Read on and you will see why gold, one of the worlds' most treasured and valuable possession's is one of the most counterfeit of commodities, something most of us have yet to discover."

*Peter Gill*

ISBN: 978-1-909424-72-2

# Contents

# Contents

# Introduction

Throughout history many claims have been made by inventors, pioneers and visionaries that have been ridiculed at the time by experts. However, years and sometimes decades later these so called experts have reluctantly had to admit they were wrong.

To give just two examples, taken from thousands, the Wright brothers could not get any journalists to witness their very first flight. This was because of a list of reasons "COMPILED BY EXPERTS" was published in the newspapers explaining why it was impossible for a heavier than air machine to be able to fly. Although this is not a political book an aspect of political history is worthy of mention. Back in 1968 the late Enoch Powell predicted that unless the doors of immigration were closed, the ever increasing ethnic minority would swamp our cities and the indigenous people would be strangers in their own country. In view of what has subsequently happened, no further comment should be necessary.

The foregoing should warn any responsible person that what we learn from the media, especially a controlled and censored one, should not be taken too seriously.

Any detective, investigative journalist, historian or researcher, who is worth their salt, will tell you that the reliability of the information they obtain is only as good as the credence of its source. If, for example, the village idiot told you that most or certain charities were just a racket to line the pockets of a few people, you would not take this claim too seriously.

However, if a similar claim was made by an accountant who had worked a number of years for some charity or other, it would or should not be dismissed so lightly. What has just been stated incidentally is just a hypothetical example and not an invective against all charities.

This is an opportune moment to say a few words about the man who was the source of information that finally resulted in this work. For reasons that will become self-evident during this exposition he prefers to be anonymous, but be assured he is by no means a    fictitious character. Indeed many people who are familiar with his work may recognise him. Throughout this book he will simply be known as Max. Now, Max was the kind of man you might read about but seldom, if ever, met.

To say that he had a diversity of hidden  talents and was knowledgeable on many subjects would be like saying that Leonardo da Vinci dabbled in oils.

Throughout his somewhat eventful life he had worked as a professional magician. This was taught to him by his father from him being seven years old. Actually, this was to stand him in good stead in later years when he became a journalist. Being a master of deception, so to speak, he was able to see through the deceptions perpetrated by governments and financial institutions on the unsuspecting public. This, among many rackets he has helped to  expose, but more about that later. He has written several books, mostly for private circulation. Suppressed history, especially  regarding the Second World War was one of his fortes. He had  interviewed many veterans from both sides and, as it is always the victors who write history books, was able to give a more balanced and accurate assessment of what had really happened and why. This was often totally different to what we have been led to believe. One secret operation that had a devastating effect on the British    economy, and a similar one that is operating at full blast at the time of writing is the topic of this book, but once again, more about this later.

Max was and probably still is, regarded by the ones who do not know him as eccentric.

He believed in fate and held the contention that there is no such thing as coincidence. According to him nothing happened by chance, every step of our life was counted and every moment measured. He enhanced his knowledge on certain aspects of occultism and esoteric topics, and especially the hidden and mystical power of numbers. Indeed among his many pursuits, for over thirty years he had practiced giving tarot and number readings and had satisfied clients from all over the world. He collected and dealt in coins, especially gold coins and was fascinated by anything counterfeit, from designer handbags to paintings, banknotes and of course coins.

The foregoing is a brief profile of Max and the source of information that has resulted in the following story. Finally, many of the names and places have been changed to protect certain individuals and governments who were and probably still are, at the time of writing, involved in a scam that would make those who committed the great train robbery look like pickpockets.

# Chapter 1

## A Passage to India

As the Airbus 330 started its descent into Goa's international airport, one of its passengers sat in excited anticipation of what this trip would have in store. Although he was reasonably well travelled this was only the second time he had visited India. The first occasion was some thirty years previously in 1981 when he was on his way to Australia. He was in Bombay for about one and a half hours when the passengers had to disembark in order for the plane to re fuel and cabin crew change. This procedure was repeated at Kuala Lumpur and Perth before completing its long haul from London to Melbourne.

This however was different; he would be spending two whole weeks with guaranteed sunshine every day. It was bitterly cold when he left Manchester and December was a good time to visit India because the monsoon season was over and he would not need an umbrella or other items to protect him from the inclement weather he had just left. However, eleven hours was a long time to be sat on a plane with little room to stretch ones legs, apart from walking or standing up in one of the isles.

During the journey he reflected on the circumstances that had prompted him to make this particular trip. It really began not long after he returned from his visit to Australia and free newspapers began to emerge. A new one was launched in the West Midlands and in the first issue there was a request for any readers who had a story to phone the editor. Max spoke to the editor and told her a little about himself. This included, among other things, that he did tarot and number readings, and was in the process of writing the second edition of one of his books. She subsequently came to see him for a consultation, was most impressed and wrote a feature about him in the next issue that generated a great deal of interest. One thing led to another and he was engaged as a special correspondent.

However his copy was so controversial that in certain quarters it went down like a lead balloon, particularly with the church and probably the establishment. Consequently, after sixteen issues, the editor, acting under instructions from her superiors, had the unpleasant task of telling him that his services were no longer required.

To some men or women this would have been a devastating blow, but not with Max. Quite the contrary as during the previous four months he had learned more about the news industry than many of his contemporaries had in as many years, and, what he had gleaned he didn't like. It was during this period that he discovered there were certain topics that were journalistic suicide to try and expose, or write about. They might get published in some local or provincial newspaper or perhaps an alternative news magazine with a small circulation, but would seldom, if ever, make the national and international press. This applied especially to what he called the medical mafia and the pharmaceutical racket. Actually he had good reason to question and doubt some doctors who many unsuspecting people entrusted their well-being and often their lives. His first wife, after being miss-diagnosed, died of cancer at the grand age of thirty five. In later years during his investigations, which included interviewing many doctors who dared not make their findings public for fear of being struck off, he discovered that many alternative remedies such as the use of certain herbs etc. we're not all quackery. This was one of the reasons he was visiting India, but we shall come to this later.

Gradually Max concluded, like many more people before him, that a controlled and mendacious media could mould people's opinions like a potter moulds his clay. As an observer of times and human nature, he also concluded that the biggest national disease, at least in the UK was apathy.

It was only when some human injustice affected an individual personally that they would protest to anybody they felt may help them to get some kind of justice. Many wrote to their MP's or newspapers only to find that their letters were ignored or they received a four line fob off. In addition to the foregoing, if this same controlled media kept telling the same blatant lies over and over again, the masses would eventually believe them. It was George Orwell who stated that 'To tell the truth in a world of deceit is a revolutionary act'. Nikita Krushev always maintained that "historians are dangerous and capable of turning everything upside down". Depending on which side you are on, both of these men were right.

Now Max had written several books and, once again, like many people before him, discovered that for every author who attained fame and fortune, thousands of talented writers went unrecognised. He himself had been writing for sixteen years before a small publisher put some of his work into print. In the earlier days of his writing he tried publishing himself but, without a proper distribution network and enough capital to finance it, he found it a very expensive pastime. Nevertheless, he wanted important information that none of the mainstream media would touch, disseminated to enlighten a few people and perhaps wake them up from their slumbered ignorance. Writing a book could take years, as has already been covered. Trying to get politicians or newspapers interested in anything that went against the status quo, would be like trying to pull a splinter our of ones backside whist wearing a boxing glove. Then, one evening, whilst listening to one of his favourite symphonies he suddenly had an idea.

He would set up his own alternative news agency. However, his next big problem was: how could this possibly be accomplished without virtually unlimited funds, which he did not have? To Max this was only a minor setback, because many years in the university of life, had taught him that the only obstacles that exist, are the ones we set up in our own minds.

One day he was browsing through a car boot sale and noticed a portable tape recorder on sale for just two pounds. After satisfying himself that it was in working order he bought it. Actually it was whilst looking at this tape recorder he suddenly realised that many programmes on the radio were recorded before being broadcast. During his career as a magician he had performed before audiences large and small and was reasonably articulate. He would produce audio presentations of hard to get information in the spoken word and market them by advertising them in alternative publications and much later on the internet. To cut a long and complex story short, over the years he had interviewed many fascinating people and got their stories on tape. These included whistle blowers from Scotland Yard, MI5, MI6, the KGB, STASI, MOSSAD, CIA and FBI and also NASA to mention a few. Some were prepared to go public but the majority preferred to remain anonymous and with good reason. One man gave Max his story and not long after met his untimely death in very dubious circumstances. Fortunately that recording is still on tape for prosperity.

Back now to why Max was in India. Max was going to interview a doctor who was an expert on Ayurvedic medicine, something that was only known by about three percent of the Indian population and probably a similar amount in the UK. The lady doctor ran a private clinic and people from all over the world came for treatment for cancer, diabetes, obesity and many other maladies. After a couple of weeks in the care of her team they returned home cured. So, interviewing this doctor coupled with a well-earned holiday in the sun was why Max was here. Little did he realise that the dice of destiny would inadvertently make him stumble on a totally different story.

Indeed, what he was to discover during the following two years or so, if made public knowledge, would rock financial institutions and the gold industry like an earthquake. But wait, I'm getting ahead of myself, let me explain how it all happened and return to the starting point of the story.

# Chapter 2

## A hairy beginning

After what seemed like an eternity his plane finally landed and came to a standstill. He had arrived. When the engines were shut down, the exit doors opened and passengers began to disembark, Max stepped into the sizzling sunshine. It felt as though he had just walked into a blast furnace after the freezing cold he had left behind in Manchester some twelve hours ago. One thing was certain; he would not need a raincoat or jersey on this trip.

During his flight he had struck up a conversation with the passenger sitting next to him, as many travellers do, especially on long haul flights. It turned out that his new acquaintance was Indian by birth but had lived in the UK for over forty years and commuted to India almost as often as Max went to Europe. His knowledge of Goa and many of its towns and villages was most extensive and it was to prove very valuable in the days that followed. He had a business that his brothers ran in Calungute.

This was quite close to the Palmarinha Hotel where Max was staying. This being the case they agreed to share a taxi to their respective destinations once they had cleared passport control, customs and immigration. This process was to take much longer than expected. A large Aeroflot plane had touched down a few minutes before them and hundreds of Russian tourists, who had come to escape their fierce winter, had crowded the somewhat small arrival hall. Furthermore there were only two officials checking passenger's passports and visas etc. Incidentally, Max had discovered some weeks previously that visiting India, at least for Brits was far from being as easy or straightforward as going to Europe, even if one had a valid passport. Indeed, the filling in of forms and other red tape, not to mention the eventual cost of about sixty pounds for a six month visa, could and had taken some four weeks.

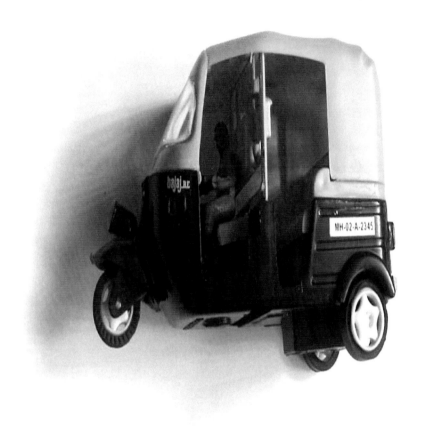

A Typical Rickshaw Taxi, similar to one that Max used.

This was due to a political 'tit for tat' measure imposed by the Indian government in retaliation for introducing more stringent conditions before allowing people from Asia, and non EU countries to enter the UK. Fortunately Max had been warned of this contingency by one of his foreign correspondents and heeded their advice. He had learned many years ago to try and profit from other peoples mistakes because a person could waste half their life learning from their own.

After standing for well over an hour waiting their turn in what was unbearable heat, they emerged from the terminal, negotiated a reasonable fare with one of the many taxi drivers, then started a drive lasting over an hour to their final destination. Just as they were getting into the taxi Rahul, Max's new companion, told him to hang onto his hat. In a matter of seconds Max, after almost having a heart attack, understood why. The driver must have passed his test, if he had ever taken one, on the wall of death or a fair ground dodgem ride. Within minutes they were driving at break neck speed on the wrong side of the road missing oncoming traffic by inches. In addition to this there were motorcycle taxis carrying some brave passengers on their pillion seat and three people riding one Lambretta scooter without a crash helmet between them, driving like lunatics. Max began to wonder what he had let himself in for and wondered if he would be reaching the safety of his hotel, let alone ever see England again. Rahul was quite used to this and  knew how to handle the situation. He offered to pay the driver an extra two hundred rupees (just over two pounds) to drive a little slower and keep on the right side of the road. Max had experienced some very hairy taxi rides in most capital cities of Europe. One of the worst was being driven round the Arc De Triumph in Paris, but nothing had equalled this journey. Incidentally, the oncoming traffic in the journey included the occasional elephant with a man sat on its back with a large stick and another man walking on in front, leading this noble beast with the aid of a rope, as though he was guiding a blind man home.  Further along the route they were sometimes held up by a herd of cows, goats or buffalo crossing the narrow roads.

At long last they reached the Palmarinha Hotel, which was en-route to Rahul's final destination. Arriving at the hotel and waiting his turn to check in, Rahul gave his new found friend a little advice. If he decided to go for a walk to familiarise himself with his new temporary environment, especially during the evening, to make sure the glass sliding doors of his apartment were firmly closed. This, Rahul explained was to prevent the likelihood of a cobra or some other snake making itself at home on or under his bed, or some other unsuspecting hiding place. With that they parted company, at least until the next day when Rahul would call for Max and give him a grand tour of the two nearby towns.

Shortly afterwards he checked in and was shown to his apartment, which was on the third floor. He tipped the porter, and lay down exhausted from the heat. Indian time is five and a half hours ahead of that in the UK. Sleeping on the plane was virtually impossible, unless one could knock themselves out with copious amounts of alcohol, usually sold at a highly inflated price on certain airlines. In a matter of minutes Max was sound asleep and did not wake up until the early evening. The very first day had been an experience that many people could have well done without and this was only the beginning.

By the way, throughout this narrative if it is stated a few times that, certain things will be explained later, it is with good reason. Complex stories, reports and situations have to be explained in a detailed step by step chronological order. This is to avoid any subsequent confusion or misunderstanding, in actual fact this is a report, which has been presented in story format in order to make it entertaining, interesting and even educational. In short, all will be revealed at the appropriate time.

# Chapter 3

## Monetary Minefields

At this stage I feel that a few words about the title of this book and some of the ramifications of this unsavoury tale are in order. There is a connection, albeit a tenuous one, with an operation executed by the Nazis code-named "Operation Bernhard" and the title of this book. Now "Operation Bernhard" which will be covered in more detail later, was an attempt by the 'German hierarchy' to disrupt or even destroy the British economy by the distribution of counterfeit banknotes during the Second World War. It also had a far more devastating effect on the economy than the British people were told a few years after the war. It must also be born in mind, and this is most important: it is always the victors who write the history books. This is not a book about coins per-se. However, "operation Midas" was and still is, at the time of this writing, an attempt to disrupt financial institutions in the West, and banks in particular, by distribution of counterfeit gold coins that would be accepted by any bullion dealer, auction house, pawnbroker and jewellers etc. without question. What is more disturbing, unlike "Operation Bernhard" which was really discovered and confirmed, and many a stable door closed after the horse had gone, so to speak, in 1944. Operation Midas is still operating at full blast and has been for at least five years. The estimated amount of counterfeit banknotes printed by "Operation Bernhard" was at least one hundred and fifty million pounds. A colossal amount in today's money, especially if one bears in mind that five pounds during the nineteen forties was often more than a week's wages. It must also be remembered that there were ten, twenty and fifty pound notes. Although they were quickly withdrawn by the Bank of England as soon as they were tipped off by the British intelligence. Nevertheless the ones that had been circulating in the meantime were honoured. In short, to put it mildly it caused an enormous headache for the Bank of England and senior officials in the currency circulation department. Incidentally the first ten pound note was re-introduced in the mid 1960's; twenty and fifty pound notes gradually came into circulation over the years that followed. In actual fact, thanks to the advance technology in printing, counterfeit banknotes have become a much bigger problem than the general public are aware, and not only in the UK. Apart from many shops and traders having special machines to detect counterfeit currency, there are plans afoot to replace the present one pound coin with a bi-metallic twelve sided one. This will be similar to the old Chamberlain brass three penny piece, so named because they were introduced by Neville Chamberlain at the beginning of the Second World War to conserve the silver that had been used to mint the old ones. It was recently stated in the mainstream media that one in three of the present pound coins in circulation are counterfeit. This is why they are probably replacing them. One pound nowadays is not much money and buys very little, but a gold sovereign, or going higher up the scale in gold coinage, a five pound piece, a US Dollar, a South African Krugerand and a fifty Mexican Peso piece are worth considerably more and are accepted as a means of exchange in all civilised countries of the world. Furthermore, certain rare historical gold coins can and often do, fetch thousands and sometimes tens of thousands at auction houses by collectors. Of course there is nothing new about any kind of fake, forgery, imitation or counterfeit depending on one's choice of words. In the course of history just about everything of value has at some time been forged or counterfeited. An Egyptian papyrus three thousand years old, now in a Stockholm museum, gave instructions on how to forge gemstones from coloured glass. The list not only includes coins, but artwork, furniture, old maps, book bindings, musical instruments, weapons, paperweights, rare stamps, snuffboxes, stock certificates, historic letters and documents, paper money, costumes and carpets, porcelain, silver candlesticks, autographs, costly watches, antique jewellery or whatever can bring a fat price in a seller's market. Or as one art dealer put it "Anything that gets expensive gets faked". We will now return to Max on that scorching December day on the Indian subcontinent, where this story really began.

# Chapter 4
## Reflection Time

The Palmarinha Hotel is roughly situated between the two towns, Mapusa and Calungute, Goa is one of the richest states in India. The hotel is really a complex comprising several shops and two outdoor swimming pools. There are two main halves or sections, one for guests and the other for people who own apartments in which they reside in or simply use as holiday homes. The whole complex is surrounded by a wall with security men guarding the two entrances. This was to prevent beggars and other unauthorised personnel disrupting the holidays of paying guests as well as the residents. There was also the possibility of a leopard or some other unwelcoming beast straying into this mini fortress during the night. This was terrifying to some unsuspecting guest who happened to fall asleep by one of the swimming pools, after a surfeit of alcohol, until the early hours of the following morning. Actually, during Max's stay, on the TV news there was a report of one man whose car had broken down in the middle of the night whilst he was driving on some desolate road. It must be remembered in many parts of India there is no street lighting, especially in rural areas. Service stations so common in the UK were few and far between. Consequently the car driver simply had to settle down in his car, fall asleep and wait until daylight . One can imagine his horror when, upon waking up, the sight that he beheld through his windscreen was a tiger fast asleep on the bonnet of his car. Fortunately, shortly after, a passing motorist pulled up beside him, frightened the beast away and came to his aid. Never the less this couldn't have done this poor man's nerves any good. There was another report, complete with video footage, of several leopards sat on the top of a hotel in Mumbai (formally Bombay) and roaming the streets. It was true that this was during the night when most people were fast asleep, but it quickly became apparent to Max that going walkabouts in certain parts of India in the early hours or after midnight was not a good idea.

This was certainly a far cry from the three, four and five star hotels where he was used to staying in Amsterdam, Munich, Madrid, Vienna and other places. Once again he began to wonder what he had let himself in for.

The first evening, after he had rested and recuperated from his perilous taxi ride, he went downstairs. The lift was about the size of a telephone box, he walked outside, sat beside one of the swimming pools and ordered a large cold beer. It seemed almost surreal sitting in shorts, wearing sandals and a sleeveless shirt in the middle of December. He reflected on the day's events, especially the long conversation he had had with Rahul during and after his flight.

Although they were from different cultures they had a great deal in common, both spiritually and philosophically. Some people might, and probably would think their ideas about the meaning of life were radical or even ridiculous. For example; both held the contention that nothing happened by chance and their meeting was no coincidence. At one point during their long in depth conversation Rahul articulated the very same thoughts that Max was actually thinking at that precise moment. Namely that every person who came into another person's life was for some specific reason which was not always apparent at the time but often became manifest days, months or even years later It was a Saturday evening on Max's first day and his appointment to interview Dr Soneta at her clinic, which has already been covered was not until the following Tuesday. This incidentally, went without a hitch. Max turned up with his tape recorder and gleaned all the information he needed about Ayurvedic medicine.

However, as this is not an exposition about the truth and benefits of herbal and other forms of alternative medicine, and has no bearing to the principle topic of this story, we will return Max's reflections by the swimming pool at the Hotel Palmamarina.

Just before retiring to his apartment for the night he received a call on his mobile phone from Rahul. The essence was that his orientation trip, to which he was looking forward, would have to be postponed until the Monday morning. This would leave Max to 'do his own thing' on Sunday. In itself this posed no problem; he was quite used to finding his own way around unfamiliar places.

He had found from his experience that the best way to gain some insight of places he was visiting was to get friendly and speak with the local people. The information to be gleaned by doing this often revealed far more important information than was printed in the attractive holiday brochures, of which we are all familiar, some of which the tour operators would rather we didn't know. This practice turned out to be priceless during the following days, as will be seen presently.  However it was growing close to bedtime and as he lay down to rest, he pondered what the following day might bring.

Had he known in advance, the investigation on which this trip would finally lead him, he would have had very little sleep.

# Chapter 5
## A Breakfast Encounter

The following morning when Max entered the breakfast room every seat was taken except for one small table for two with one empty place. The other was occupied by a fairly attractive fair haired lady in her early forties, reading a German magazine. It was a buffet bar where one simply helped themselves to whatever took their fancy. Carrying a plate with two croissants in one hand and a cup of coffee in the other, he walked over to the table in question and asked the lady if he could join her. She nonchalantly looked up at him, then to her left and right and seeing there were no other spaces available, nodded in assent and carried on reading. Whilst he was eating and drinking his coffee he noticed an ashtray with several cigarette stubs alongside a half empty packet of cigarettes. It must be remembered that this was India where draconian laws on smoking in public did not apply as they do in Europe. It was quite obvious that this lady, like Max, for all his sins, was quite a heavy smoker. After he had finished eating he asked her in German if she objected to him smoking. She looked up, gave him a quizzical look, and put her magazine down, after telling Max she didn't mind and went on to light up a cigarette herself. Now Max, apart from being a shrewd observer of times, could deduce a great deal from the way people spoke, their body language, how they dressed and many other things from their general demeanour that would probably go unnoticed by the average person. It was this facet of his character that made him so good at his profession. At the same time he was very trusting and treated any human being as a possible friend until their actions proved them to be selfish, scheming or even treacherous. When this lady put her magazine down on the table he noticed it was open at the horoscope page. Quite casually he asked her, in English, if she had been reading what her stars foretold. She just smiled and said she only read them for amusement and that astrology and similar beliefs should not be taken seriously.

Whilst they were engrossed in casual conversation, he noticed a gold coin in a setting that she was wearing around her neck as a kind of pendant. Although it intrigued him, for some reason he could not account for at the time, he kept his thoughts to himself. Throughout their brief small talk he learned that she loved to travel, was very fond of nature, especially botany, loved painting and anything aesthetic and much more. Just as he was getting up to leave he casually asked her if her birth sign was Sagittarius and if she was born on the seventh or sixteenth of December. This really took her back. Looking somewhat surprised and nodding her head she asked him how he could possibly have known or even guessed such a thing. To this he simply replied that sometimes he was a good guesser and that if or when she had an hour to spare he would     explain. . With that he bade her farewell and thought no more about the matter. Sometimes, a woman's curiosity and intuition knows no bounds. The lady in question, who we will call Frau Schreiber, had a very enquiring nature and had no intention whatever of letting the flippant comment of her new acquaintance rest. Indeed, she made up her mind to satisfy her curiosity as soon as the opportunity presented itself. Max of course was completely oblivious of this at the time.

The rest of the day he spent by one of the swimming pools, enjoying the sunshine and talking to some of the other guests and hotel employees. It was from the latter, who were eager to talk to this Englishman who showed such an interest in their country, that he learned more about the customs, poverty, corruption and political administration in a single day than the average tourist would in one month. His first shock was that an average wage was the equivalent of thirty five pounds per month. He quickly realised that every time he gave one of the staff an English pound coin as a tip, he had given what was to them a day's wages. Little wonder he became popular during his stay.

The people, who for whatever reason, could not or would not work for such a pittance, would have to beg on the streets or starve. If one had the misfortune to fall ill or get injured and could not pay for proper medical care they died. There was no welfare system which the British take so much for granted, in spite of its flaws and incompetence. It was common knowledge in the west that the vast sums of money given to third world countries as aid never usually reached the people for whom it was intended. Every government, local, national or federal has its share of corrupt officials but how so few people in high positions could reduce so many to poverty in what was after all a wealthy country disturbed him. Worse still, if any tourist reported a crime, especially theft, which was quite common, to the police, Rupees would have to exchange hands. Hundreds or thousands of rupees were to be paid or nothing would happen. There was one member of staff, a waiter, with whom Max became very friendly, and who was a mine of information. Amongst other things, he learned that there used to be, a few years ago, many German tourists who came to Goa and were not very popular. However over a period of time they were gradually replaced by Russians who were even more unpopular. Indeed the local people would have welcomed back the Germans with open arms, and with good reason. The Indian government had recently amended its property laws so that any foreigners who wanted to buy land, houses or hotels etc. would have to be married to, or have a partner who was domicile in India. This, it was explained, was to put a halt to the equivalent of the Russian Mafia from continuing to buy property or businesses. Thus, getting a toe hold that could eventually become a stranglehold on the economy and the country itself. Max secretly thought that this would be an ideal policy for the British Government to introduce. Over the years one industry and institution after another has been sold to any foreigners who had the money to buy it. So much so that when one buys virtually anything in the UK and for that matter gets a job, the average person hasn't a clue who they are actually buying from, or who they work for.

It had been quite a day and an education, but it was the following day when he learned, first hand, that his waiter friend knew what he was talking about.

## Chapter 6
## Russian Revelations

Rickshaw taxis are a common means of transport in India. In actual fact one does not have to travel so far to experience the uncomfortable ride in one of these three wheeled monstrosities. They have been imported to Totnes in Devon and are quite popular with the tourists for their novelty and the owners for their economy. Why? Because the fuel upon which the car runs on is cooking oil, probably re-cycled, and only costs about three pounds per week to run. Be that as it may, at ten thirty the following morning Rahul called for Max in one of these vehicles and they embarked on another perilous journey to a nearby town called Mapusa. After what seemed like an eternity, but was only about half an hour with Max being on the verge of a nervous breakdown, they arrived at their destination and parked next to a row of motorcycles and scooters. The owner of the taxi incidentally, was a good friend of Rahul's who, like many of these wretched people, was just trying to make an honest living with the limited facilities available to him and at his disposal. After clambering out of this excuse of a car and narrowly missing stepping into a large cowpat in the road, they parted company with the driver for a couple of hours and made their way to the market. As they walked along and Max was drinking in the scene that lay before his eyes, he felt as though he was on another planet. There were no traffic lights, pedestrian crossings or litter bins, cows wandered performing their natural functions unhindered on the roads, pavement or any place they chose. It was quite common to see them asleep by cars or motorcycles and it goes without saying   India is one of the few places in the world (or was at least at this time) where you do not see the ubiquitous Mc Donald's, There was every conceivable kind of rubbish strewn everywhere.

Beggars and homeless people were sat and sometimes sleeping on pavements. One sight almost moved him to tears and will be forever etched in his memory till his dying day. There was a man, probably in his forties, with no legs, just a couple of stumps, on a board, about two feet square with a wheel at each corner pushing himself along with the aid of a short stick begging. As they meandered through the market what he had just seen reminded him of what the Arabs used to say: "I complained I had no shoes till I saw a man with no feet". He also thought that it would do people good in the UK to visit India and see it first hand, which is totally different to watching it on TV. They might then appreciate, in spite of a controlled media and corrupt or depraved politicians, how fortunate they really were and should be truly thankful.

Rahul introduced Max to a trader friend of his who had a shop in the market that sold clothes and fabrics. He was in a terrible mood and with good reason as about to be explained. He showed Rahul a hundred Russian Rouble banknote that had been tendered by one of the many Russian tourists. However, when he took it to the bank, along with several others, the bank would not accept them as they were counterfeit, albeit good ones that would fool most people; they had even got the right watermark. Max bought the note from him for one hundred rupees (just over one pound) as an interesting memento. Then, to his astonishment this unfortunate trader asked him if he wanted anymore, opened his wallet and revealed a wedge of them. Heaven knows how much this poor man and many other honest traders were cheated in this way. Max began to realise why the locals would welcome back the Germans with open arms. But, human nature, being what it is, there are always a few who spoil things for the many. By this time the heat had become overbearing and he implored his friend to take him back to the sanctuary of the hotel.

Whilst they were driving along he was informed about another disturbing incident that seemed unbelievable. There was a Russian tourist who shot a taxi driver dead over some dispute over the fare. Far from the culprit being arrested and sent to jail, he simply paid the police and the family of the victim a substantial sum of money and was allowed to return to his homeland like any other tourist. During the evening Max was sitting on the outdoor terrace with a drink minding his own business and reflecting on the day's events. Whilst he was deep in thought he felt a gentle tap on the shoulder, caught a whiff of perfume, turned round and saw his breakfast acquaintance of the previous morning. It was Frau Schreiber who asked him if she could join him. It had already been quite a day for him but he was soon to learn it was far from over.

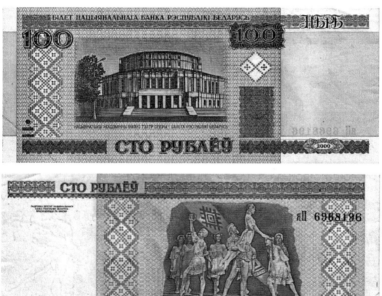

Thousands of these counterfeit 100 Rouble notes were circulated in certain parts of India, especially Goa. They caused considerable financial distress with traders, and have since been withdrawn

# Chapter 7
## Fate & Fortune

Before he had the chance to answer she promptly sat herself down at his table, beckoned a waiter and asked Max what he wanted to drink. This was something he wasn't used to and at that precise moment was not particularly welcome. However, not wishing to be rude and with as much politeness and diplomacy he could muster, he said that a fresh pineapple juice would suffice. He also perceived that he could say goodbye to his early night.

At this point it must be born in mind that for over thirty years he had done thousands of number, tarot and sometimes palm readings for people, mostly women, from all walks of life. During this period he had developed his intuition to a degree that many detectives would envy. Indeed, sometimes when he was in close company with someone he could read their thoughts, which were often totally different from the words that came out of their mouths. At times it was embarrassing for him and would have been most disconcerting for the individual had they been aware of this whilst in his company.

In anticipation of what was going to follow he felt the best means of defence was attack. To this end, and before Ingrid, which was her christian name, had the opportunity to bombard him with questions, he quickly asked her one.

His eyes could sometimes be quite penetrating and, looking straight into her eyes he asked her to think of someone she knew very well who he could not possibly know and just tell him the persons birthday and if the person was still alive. After a few moments of thinking she gave him the birthday of a man she knew very well but had since passed away.

To her utter astonishment he not only gave a most accurate assessment of his character and how he made a living, but also his age date and day of the week he probably died. All of which was correct except the birth sign of his wife or partner, who was still alive. Pausing for a drink to allow what he had just told her to sink in, he then followed up with something else she wasn't expecting. However, this was after shaking her head, either in disbelief or astonishment, probably the latter, at what was imparted, she jokingly remarked that it was a good thing they were not living in the middle ages. Had this been the case, he would most certainly have been tried, convicted and executed for being in a league with the devil.

Max then explained that in those days, as now, there were and still are double standards: one for the poor and ignorant, and another for the rich, powerful and enlightened. Throughout the ages such people, especially the hierarchy of the church and certain secret societies, have supressed vital esoteric information from the masses by means of fear, death or ridicule. Incidentally, this also applied to magicians, adept in legerdemain or sleight of hand, who travelled with other players to towns and fairs. Many of these harmless entertainers were tortured and put to death unless they revealed the secrets of their sorcery.

Apart from students of occultism, most academies, universities and other places of great learning could have no means of knowing that some of the greatest kings in the world owed their success and wealth to advice given by these astrologers. Only the Egyptian magicians had greater power than priests or potentates. They had perhaps never read that Queen Elizabeth 1 consulted her astrologer Dr John Dee on all important matters of state and that the destiny of England had been guided by those students of occultism whom they were taught were but fit companions for black cats and were workers of the devil.

They perhaps had never heard of that great English astrologer William Lilly, who predicted the fire of London fifteen years before it took place, or that the House of Commons had called him before that great assembly believing that as he had predicted the calamity with such accuracy, he could explain what had caused such a catastrophe.

Further, their English history had never taught them that Charles 1 had given the first thousand pounds his government had, sent to the same Lilly, the astrologer, asking him to predict his fate, and that had the King taken heed of the warnings given to him by the astrologer he might never have lost his head and descended into posterity as Charles the martyr. Again, it is predictable they never knew that Queen Anne maintained an occultist in the roll of the Privy Purse, and that she had such faith in the celebrated Van Galgebrok, that she asked him to predict the year of her death. This he did with perfect accuracy three years before the event, which took place on August 1$^{st}$ 1714.

Max then casually mentioned that he himself could cite cases from his own career when he had predicted the date of many people's deaths years before they occurred, but quickly added that he no longer did this because most people would not thank him for telling them when their number was up, so to speak. At this point Max yawned, drained his glass, stood up and told Ingrid that he was very tired and was turning in. However by this time, Frau Schreiber had no intention of letting him go so easily.

Although she couldn't make up her mind whether to fear or respect him, she was now of the firm opinion that he certainly knew what he was talking about. She stood up, caught his hand and asked how much he would charge her for a consultation. Max gave her a kindly smile, shook his head and told her that he no longer practiced because there were certain things many people were better off not knowing. She was insistent however and said that everyone had a price of some kind, what was his?

He was about to tell her that he couldn't be bought when his eyes rested on the gold coin in the pendant she was wearing. Almost in desperation to get away and to his bed he asked her if she would consider selling him the pendant round her neck. To his utter astonishment she promptly removed it, thrust it in his hands telling him it was a gift if he would oblige her. Instead he accepted, agreed to her request and arranged a consultation the following evening in her apartment. Had Max realised what a Pandora's Box he was about to open, he would have thrust it back into her well-manicured hands and caught the next available plane back to the UK.

# Chapter 8
## A woman's mouth is a deep pit, be careful not to fall therein

Although there have been many women in Max's life, mostly platonic, it must be emphatically stated he was by no means a lothario or woman chaser. He enjoyed the company of the opposite sex, and they his, but he firmly believed that friendships were better and usually lasted far longer than an affair. Indeed in spite of many opportunities that had come his way, he held the view that it was cruel to cross the Rubicon or enter into a physical relationship unless he genuinely cared for the lady in question.

It might have been his imagination but he thought that Frau Ingrid Schreiber had displayed a little more interest than was usual for a prospective client who simply wanted her fortune told. Generally speaking it was one of three things that concerned those who availed themselves of his services: Money, health or some relationships. Ingrid was certainly not poor and seemed quite healthy. It was true she wore no wedding ring, but a woman with her looks and personality must have had, or may still have many admirers. Why should she make a gift of something so seemingly valuable for a service she could so easily obtain from one of the local mystics or seers, for just a few hundred rupees? At the same time he was also aware that appearances could be very deceptive.

He had learned over the years that many people carried some secret burden in their hearts. They had possibly been guided by fate or instantly felt he was a man in whom they could safely confide. Indeed, had Max chosen to go with the blackmail business he could have been a millionaire several times over.

During his mental meanderings it suddenly occurred to him that he hadn't got his tarot cards, which had been on a shelf gathering dust for years. After his experience in Mapusa, going into the nearest town to try and buy some without Rahul as his guide and escort, was about as appealing as going nude hand gliding in the Himalayas. However this did not pose a real problem. Being a magician he always carried a few small props with him on his travels, these included a few packs of cards. Actually the latter  always reminded him of poem by Chesterton entitled "Magic" part of it which ran:

> "I have a hat but not to wear
> I wear a sword but not to slay
> And ever in my bag I bear
> A pack of cards but not to play"

Strange to say, most magicians seldom play cards. They regard them as an important, even sacred tool of their craft. Also the suits of clubs, hearts, spades and diamonds of conventional playing cards are derived from the suites of batons, cups, swords and coins of the tarot. It is also true that there are two packs in the tarot known as the major and minor arcana. The former comprises twenty two major trumps and is not included in the packs most people play with. However, there is one card from the greater arcana which often is "The Fool", more commonly known as the joker. For this reason anyone who fully understands all this and much more, and knows exactly what they are doing, the practise of Cartomancy, or fortune telling by playing cards, can be just as accurate as using the tarot. The foregoing is just to give the reader a brief understanding of what is being gradually unfolded.

Max turned up at her apartment at the appointed time, knocked on the door, was shown in and offered a drink from a large bottle of wine, which he accepted, and was led to her balcony. Ingrid looked absolutely beautiful. She was wearing a pale blue dress that clung, revealing the contours of her perfect figure. The smell of the perfume that assailed his nostrils shortly after his arrival almost intoxicated him.

As they sat down facing each other at the table on that warm December evening with not even a breeze, he secretly wondered what she could possibly want with or from him; after all, he was old enough to be her father. Whilst sipping his wine and Ingrid was lighting up a cigarette he recalled one of his clients, several years ago telling him that she would rather be an older man's darling than a younger man's slave. It has always been by no means uncommon for young women to marry older men and vice versa. However, Max was not in the market for romance. Indeed, in his experience he had learned the hard way that some of the most attractive women he had known turned out to be the most lethal.

In short, although this charming and vivacious lady had done him no harm at this stage, he was on his guard in case this incident turned out to be some kind of tender trap. He then got down to the purpose of their meeting. Max explained that every practitioner in his particular field had their own way of working, and he was no exception. His methods were unorthodox and may be considered by some as reprehensible, but ultimately in his client's interest. Placing his portable tape recorder on the table he further explained, that he recorded his readings because most of his clients would not be able to remember everything they were told.

Consequently when the tape was given to them after the consultation they could play it, if or when they chose and thus have something to which they could refer. It was the reading of her cards which is relevant to this story so this is what will be outlined. Before asking her to shuffle the cards etc. he asked her to mentally ask them what she wanted them to tell her. He then cautioned her warning that sometimes it could be like opening a Pandora's box, which was one reason he had ceased practicing. Rather like Prospero in Shakespeare's mystical play The Tempest. Part of one of his speeches ran:

> "But this rough magic I here abjure
> I'll break my staff
> Bury it certain fathoms in the earth
> And deeper than did plummet sound
> I'll drown my book"

He also told her that the answer or answers which the cards gave was sometimes what the person was hoping or praying for, but could also be what they were not expecting or even dreading. Either way he would tell her. After he had gone through the procedure which he had done thousands of times with people form all walks of life, he gave her an assessment of what the cards told him, which was as follows: First of all she had no health or financial problems. Quite the contrary, whatever else she might have to contend with, health and money worries would not be one of them. However, on the emotional plain things were not and never would be what she had hoped for. She was at a crossroads in her life and would have to make an important decision very soon. It concerned a choice between two men in her life. The first was someone who was much older than her. He was highly intelligent and probably an academic such as a lawyer, teacher, lecturer or even some kind scientist. At this point Ingrid almost choked on her drink. The man, Max continued, was very successful but did not hoard his success to himself. He was very kind and compassionate and would never refuse a person any help that was within his power to give. Although he held, and always would hold a special place in her heart, he was no longer in her life in the conventional way, possibly due to the geographical distance between them. The second man, he continued, was much younger than her self and of a poetic and reflective nature and very understanding. Also he was devoted to her as she was to him, but he was poor and without any prospects of keeping her in the way to which she had become accustomed.

In a nutshell she was going to have to choose one or the other of these men, but whatever choice she made would entail some considerable sacrifice on her part. By this time Ingrid had con-sumed almost half the bottle of wine and was getting a little tipsy, she asked Max which one she should choose and would she be happy, to which he replied that he could only answer that question after she had decided for herself exactly what or who she wanted. He further pointed out that with the best will in the world people like him could only do so much. It was true that certain events in one's life were set in stone which nothing could alter, but to a large extent we and our lives were the result of some decision or decisions we had taken at some time or another. If she really wanted to know and decided, it would mean a second reading and may be necessary for him to look in her hands, but not at that particular moment as it was getting late.

For some reason he suddenly felt sorry for her and reaching into his pocket, handed back to her the gift she had thrust into his hand the previous evening, explaining that it was far too generous for the service he had just rendered. She promptly put it back in his hand and told him it was only a cheap piece of imitation gold jewel-lery she had bought on one of the many bazaars. With that they parted company and Max returned to his apartment, after he had reluctantly agreed to see her again the following evening.

Just before going to bed he carefully extracted the coin from its setting. He examined it very closely with the aid of his jeweller's glass. Within a few minutes he realised that what he held up in his hands was no cheap gold plated trinket. Judging from its weight and feel it was either perfectly genuine, in which case worth about two thousand pounds, or the best counterfeit he had ever seen or handled. Over the years hundreds of fake coins had passed through his hands but he had never seen anything like the one he was holding. It gradually became apparent there was something about Frau Schreiber that wasn't quite right. Exactly what it was he knew not, but he was determined to find out.

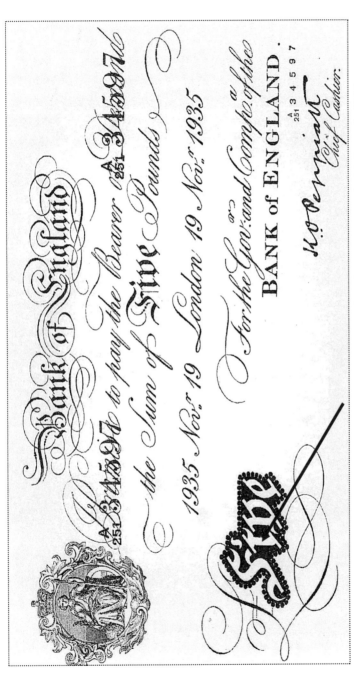

The above Bank notes were first issued by the Bank of England in 1793 and withdrawn in 1956

Note the slight glitch in the letter I in the word FIVE. This was deliberately inserted to detect forgeries

Even this was not overlooked in Operation Bernhard.

## Chapter 9
## A Monetary Interlude

Before proceeding any further I feel that an explanation of why Max was so excited about his recent acquisition from Frau Schreiber. To this end, although this is not meant to be some kind of numismatists or coin collections guide, a few words about this hobby or profession are necessary to give the layman a brief    insight as to how and why some  coins are more valuable than   others to collectors.

Many people are under the erroneous impression that because a coin is very old it is valuable. Although this is true in some cases, it is not, and should not be used as a yardstick for valuation purposes. The two principle factors that determine the value of coins is their condition and scarcity. This applies to the ones made of copper or tin, as well as silver or gold. Another false notation harboured by the layman is that low denomination coins are of little value, Allow me to give two hypothetical examples to illustrate what I mean.

Just suppose you had a George the third golden guinea that was minted in 1797 and was left to you in the will of your late Aunt Fanny. If it was almost worn flat through constant circulation it would only be worth the value of the gold it contained, which varies from day to day. On the other hand, if it was in very good condition with every detail plainly visible and had not been bent or defaced in any way, it could be worth several hundred or even a few thousand pounds. The second example, although hypothetical, is not as farfetched as it may seem. Indeed a very similar experience happened to Max. Suppose you were fortunate enough to pick up a Queen Anne farthing in very good condition for a couple of pounds at a car boot or jumble sale.

If anyone wanted to buy this same coin the price tag would be around the five hundred pounds mark, and anyone who doubts or denies this statement should try buying one from any reputable coin dealer. In view of the foregoing it should go without saying that collecting or dealing in these pieces of metal is a highly specialist pastime or profession. Furthermore it can also be very costly; especially if one buys some valuable item which they subsequently discover is counterfeit.

Now what Max had become so curious or even excited about was a James the Second golden guinea in beautiful condition, even if it were a counterfeit. King James the Second, the younger brother of Charles the Second, reigned from 1685 until 1688 until he was defeated or usurped by William of Orange, later to become William the Third. To go into the history of the monarchy would be far too much digression. However, if one considers the logistics of the above statement it must be obvious, even to the simplest of people, that the shorter reign of a monarch, especially over three hundred years ago, the scarcer the coins, minted at the time, have become. It must also be remembered, and should logically follow, that coins minted during the reigns of George the Third and Queen Victoria, who were on the throne for over sixty years, are far more plentiful. In short, as the title of a previous chapter stated: this particular profession can be a monetary minefield. Now let's return back to the Palmarinha Hotel and Max's new investigation.

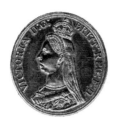

British £5 Jubilee piece 1887

Counterfeit

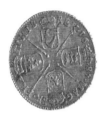

James the second Golden
Guinea 1687.

The best counterfeit coin
Max had ever seen, this
was passed as genuine by
many experts and started
his investigation. See
chapters 8 and 13

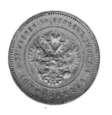

Russian 37.5 Roubles 1907

Counterfeit

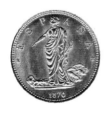

Spain 100 Pesetas 1870

Counterfeit

# Chapter 10
## A Waiters Tale

The following day whilst he was sitting by one of the swimming pools he spotted his waiter friend and beckoned him to come over. We will call this waiter Baba.

That particular day happened to be his day off and, like most of the employees, had their own accommodation on the premises. Their scanty wages did not allow them to have very much, if any, social life. Consequently he was more than happy when Max asked him to join him for a drink or two, especially in view of the generous tips he had been receiving. During their conversation Max casually asked him if he knew anything about one of their patrons, Frau Schreiber. His companion shook his head and told Max that he knew very little, she had been coming here every year about the same time for about three years, and largely kept herself to herself. Then looking furtively to his left and right, he whispered that what she spent on drink throughout her stay was more than he could earn in two months. She was obviously a woman of means.

Without seeming too inquisitive and making this meeting like an interrogation, he once more asked quite causally, after ordering his friend another drink, if she ever had any visitors. Now, human nature, being what it is, makes it surprising what a person can recall when their memories are jogged. Indeed, sometimes hearing a piece of music, having a glass of wine or even being shown a photograph can evoke certain events in a person's life which they thought was long forgotten. In this case, once again his friend shook his head and said only on one occasion, which was the previous year.

She had been there for a few days and was joined by a German gentleman who remained and shared her apartment for the rest of her stay. When asked, once again quite casually, if he remembered anything about the gentleman such as his age and so on, his waiter friend replied that he certainly did. He sat back and, for a few moments, seemed to be in a world of his own re-living some pleasant occasion. Rather like someone recalling their first holiday or first love. At length he said it was difficult to guess because he was grey haired but could have been in his fifties or early sixties. Whatever his age, he was quite distinguished and most gracious and polite as well as being very kind. The reason he remembered him so vividly was because whilst this gentleman was checking in at the reception, he had overheard a conversation that Baba was having with his boss in the corner of the foyer. The essence of which was that Baba was asking for an advance on his wages for medical treatment for his mother, treatment which was urgently needed. His request was politely but firmly denied and Baba resumed his duties looking very despondent. However, this new guest followed him out into the courtyard and asked him how much he needed. Looking rather puzzled he said a lot of money, three thousand Rupees (just over thirty pounds), Almost one month's wages. To Baba's utmost astonishment this stranger opened his wallet and thrust four thousand Rupees into his hand, and even before he had chance to thank him he went back to reception to resume his checking in process. He was hoping to be greeted by Frau Schreiber but she was not there. It turned out she was fast asleep, probably as a result of a copious amount of alcohol. As can be imagined Baba was eternally grateful and throughout this gentleman's stay, he went out of his way to cater for his every need .

Strange to say that in spite of his affluence, what this kind gentleman needed was someone sympathetic, to whom he could open his heart to, and confide.

Max fully understood this as he himself had been a combination of a counsellor, priest, psychiatrist and confidante to thousands of people for many years.

Over the following few days Baba learned that Ulrich, the gentleman's name, was from the British sector of West Berlin but some years previously he had re-located to some country in the Middle East due to his work which he said was a kind of specialist in metals. Frau Schreiber had been his girlfriend for many years. They had met not long after her divorce, became an item and were very happy. However since the collapse of communism a number of things had occurred that had prompted him to leave. He did not like what was happening in Germany and Berlin in particular, there were as many Turks living there as Germans. The whole country, if not Europe itself, was becoming a multiracial Babylon.

Then one day, as what was said in that famous film: "The Godfather" someone made him an offer he couldn't refuse. It entailed him going to live in a different country, but that was no hardship to him. He thought Frau Schreiber would be over the moon and jump at the chance. Unfortunately she did not share his enthusiasm and would not leave her native Germany, except for holidays. Eventually a compromise was reached and she agreed to give it a try for three months while she remained in Berlin, fully confident that he would be glad to be back in as many weeks. She turned out to be wrong,

Trial separations are not always a good idea because they often have a habit of becoming permanent with one or the other person becoming bitter and regretting such an agreement.

The thing Baba recalled so vividly was that Ulrich never tired of and enjoyed talking about his grandmother, what a grand old lady she was. Her mind was as sharp as a razor right up to the day she died well into her nineties. Actually it was shortly before her death when he received the offer he could not refuse, and firmly believed she was helping him on the other side. Unfortunately, since he had parted from Frau Schreiber, they only met occasionally whilst she was on holiday in a warmer climate. Like Russia the German winters can be very severe, and she had become an alcoholic. He missed good German beer but he could take it or leave it. This applied to most things in his life including women and was possibly one of the reasons he never married,

By this time the sun was really beginning to burn Max badly, so they parted company. But It had been a most informative meeting.

# Chapter 11
## Liquor, Loose Lips and the Nazi Connection

It is common practice for many detectives to trick suspects into making a confession, by pretending to know more than they actually do. If they have a few scraps of information which they know is true this increases their chance of success. On a similar plain but for different and less favourable motives, certain unscrupulous pseudo psychics, mediums, clairvoyants etc. use this modus operandi to convince their unsuspecting and often desperate and gullible clients that they are as genuine as they claim to be. This is largely achieved by getting a one or more of their accomplices to make a few discreet enquiries about their prospective clients.

Max abhorred this practice but in this particular case he felt that the end justified the means. One must also not lose sight of the fact that he was a master of deception and such an undertaking to him would be child's play, as it turned out to be. Armed with this unexpected but most welcome intelligence, that evening he knocked on the door of Frau Schreiber's apartment once more. He felt as quietly confident as a poker player holding a royal flush, the only hand that cannot be beaten. When Ingrid, as she insisted on being called, greeted him, she looked as lavishing as she had on the previous evening, but already tipsy. Once more they went on to the balcony and sat down at the small table on another breezeless night. Max put his portable tape recorder and cards down and was ready to begin. Whilst she was pouring him a drink, he suddenly decided to start, by using an old and fairly common strategy used very often by charlatans and magicians alike.

In psychic terminology this is called psychometry. A genuine  psychometrist asks his client for some object which he or she holds in their hand or sometimes holds it on the centre of their forehead, they are then able to tell their client where it came from, who it belonged to and lots of other information which can be enlightening, embarrassing and sometimes incriminating. Indeed, the police often used such people in solving certain crimes, especially murder cases, although they seldom admit this to the public.

To this end, Max asked Ingrid if she could give him something, preferably metal, that was given to her by one of her gentleman friends. This, he explained, was for him to hold in order to see if he could pick up any vibration, and give some kind of insight into the person it came from. She then went to her large handbag and after fishing through the contents, gave him a beautiful cameo brooch in a gold setting. Just before Max put it to his forehead and pretended to concentrate, he perceived that it was quite old and originally belonged to an elderly person. His next step was going to be a gamble, but he took it. After pretending to concentrate for a few moments he asked her if the name Ulrich meant anything. She looked a little startled and told him it was the name of the man who gave her the brooch. He then quickly followed by asking if this man had a close affinity with his grandmother. Upon hearing the word grandmother she almost went berserk and launched into a frenzied tirade against the woman so much revered by Ulrich.

That woman, she almost screamed, was one of the most evil people who ever lived. She was an unrepentant fanatical Nazi to her dying day. Were it not for her insane dreams and misguided ideology, Ulrich and she would still be living happily together in her beloved Germany. She was the former mistress of a man who should have been tried and hanged at the Nuremburg trials. He must have been born under a lucky star, because he managed to slip through the ever enclosing net that was encircling him by the allies. If that were not enough, apart from managing to get to South America with a passport supplied by the Vatican, he had accrued   enough money from his nefarious activities to spend the rest of his life in indolent luxury. Furthermore, Ilsa, Ulrich's grand-mother, did not have to live and endure the poverty, shortage of food and many other privations of post war Germany like millions of others. Thanks to her lovers money and expertise in financial machinations, she was able to take the bastard son she had born him, (Ulrich's father) and live in Switzerland until Germany was get-ting back on its feet, only then did she return. By this time Ingrid was almost spitting sparks and breathing fire, Max motioned with his free hand to calm down before she burst a blood vessel and asked her to pour him another drink. Whilst she was so doing he falsely told her that information from the brooch he was holding was coming to him thick and fast. However, before he was pre-pared to enlarge on this it was necessary to ask her one more im-portant question to which she must answer truthfully. Otherwise he could be of no further service if she really wanted him to put her mind and anxiety at rest.

When Ingrid asked what the question was, Max placed the placed the coin that he had carefully removed from its setting, that she had previously given him, on the table. He looked her straight in the eye and asked her how she came by it. He quickly added that she was not to repeat the fairy story she had previously given about having bought it in some bazaar. She went silent and looked very deep in thought, finally she said that even if she told him he would never believe her. To which Max replied, "Try me". First of all she asked him to switch off his tape recorder, which he did. She then said she that she needed another drink and almost staggered into the kitchen of her apartment for another bottle of wine to replace the empty one on the table. During her brief absence Max dis-creetly switched the tape back on again and placed it out of imme-diate sight. It had a very sensitive microphone and could still pick up a conversation within a range of a few feet, providing there was no background noise or loud music. By now Ingrid was quite intoxi-cated but they say that a drunken man (or woman) often speaks  a sober mind. In view of this old but truthful adage he just sat back and let her prattle on, only interrupted by short intervals when she lit another cigarette or replenished her large glass.

The topics she rambled on about for the best part of an hour were many. They included right wing politics, biochemistry, alchemy, senior former Nazi officials, replica gold and counterfeit currency. Incidentally, to substantiate her claim and probably convince Max she was telling the truth, she once more staggered into her lounge and started rummaging in her large handbag. She returned and slammed half a dozen of what appeared to be gold coins on the table. Even though she was quite drunk she could see by the expression on his face that he was most impressed as well as surprised. This seemed to sober her up and she stood stiffly to at-tention. But suddenly, she asked to be excused to use the toilet, after all she joked, one only rented what they were drinking.

Whilst she was absent he realized that the tape on his recorder had run out some time ago. He then quietly replaced it with another and put the one that had the recording on in his pocket. Turning it over and spooling it back was too fiddly and Ingrid could return at any moment, so replacing it was more expedient. When she did return to the table there was an air of confidence about her, almost smugness. Acting as nonchalantly and casually as if she was offering someone a cigarette, with a wave of her hand she said he could keep what she had just put on the table. They were to her; she went on, a mere trifle as she could get dozens or even hundreds like them if she wanted. However she would like something from him in return, in addition to the continuation of her reading. When Max asked what it was she leaned across the table, looked him straight in the eye and pointed to his tape recorder. She wanted the tape he had secretly been recording. Frau Schreiber was not as intoxicated as she appeared.

Acting with simulated resignation Max removed the cassette from his machine and handed it over. His heart was beating like a drum as he hoped and prayed that she wouldn't ask for it to be played back. She would then discover it was a blank and that Max had tried to fool her yet again. Fortunately she didn't, but simply pulled yards and yards of tape out of the cassette until it looked as though she was holding a ball of string. She then flung it as hard and far away from her balcony as she possibly could, and a few seconds later they both heard a little splash. It had obviously landed in one of the swimming pools.

By this time Max was beginning to feel a little uncomfortable in her company. Re-gaining his composure he proceeded to deal out his cards he told her what she had in her hearts of hearts and already knew and was expecting. Nevertheless she was more than satisfied even though it was not what she had hoped to hear. Max then looked at his watch and standing up he gathered his cards along with the coins, barely giving them a second glance. He placed them in his bag along with his tape recorder and, after thanking Ingrid for her hospitality and an interesting evening bade her goodnight.

It was an experience and its aftermath he would remember for a long time. However, for the moment he decided to put the entire incident out of his mind and enjoy the rest of his holiday, which he did.

On his return flight to Manchester Max would have the time and the inclination to reflect, review and analyse everything that occurred between himself and his recent German acquaintance.

## Chapter 12
"When you eliminate the impossible whatever you have left no matter how improbable, is the truth" - Sherlock Holmes.

Long haul flights, even with many a seasoned traveller is an experience to which they seldom look forward to. Once upon a time travel by air was a pleasant and even exciting adventure. One could look forward to excellent complimentary food and drinks. Although these and other perks are still to be had on certain airlines without the passengers having to pay through the nose, they are becoming increasingly few. On this particular trip, which was a package holiday, the food on each flight was thrown in, but according to many passengers it should have been thrown out. In short, travel by air in the twenty first century can be a veritable nightmare. When he was about two hours into the flight back to the UK, he realised that many of his fellow passengers were using laptops and various other electronic gizmos. Now for all Max's talents, when it came to operating some of the modern gadgets, which most youngsters find quite easy, he was out of his depth. So much so, that when travelling, he preferred to carry an old Walkman and a few tapes in his hand luggage. It never bothered him when he sometimes got a few strange looks, providing he could listen to some of his favourite symphonies and other music in peace. It was whilst he was looking in his bag that he noticed the tape recording he made during his encounter with Ingrid Schreiber, but he had put it out of his mind to enjoy the rest of his holiday. As he had nothing to do, and several hours of time on his hands he decided to play the drunken or seemingly drunken invective delivered against poor Ulrich's grandmother. Unfortunately many of the people she maligned were dead and therefore unable to defend themselves. Even if only half of what she claimed was true, it would make anything written by Ian Fleming, the creator of James Bond stories, pale into insignificance.

The Following is a brief summary:

First of all the lover of Ulrich's grandmother was a man called Friedrich Schwend. He was married but it was not uncommon for married men to confide more in their mistresses than they do with their wives. During their relationship she bore him a son, Ulrich's father. Friedrich Schwend was one of the key men, if not one of the most important, in the distribution of counterfeit British Banknotes in a Nazi scam called Operation Bernhard. (This has already been briefly outlined in chapter three.) Throughout his career with the Nazis and before he fled to South America, he managed to accumulate a considerable fortune. This was accomplished through the discreet purchase of gold, precious stones and antiques etc. All of which were paid for with counterfeit British banknotes. Once more, he discreetly converted these items into liquid assets and hard currency such as U.S. dollars. The dollar it must be remembered, at that time was very strong and not on the point of collapse as it has been since. He put a considerable amount of this money into various bank accounts in Sweden, Switzerland, Portugal and other neutral countries, not to mention into wise investments.

This enabled him to get Ilsa, and her bastard son, ensconced in Switzerland with an income on which it would be possible for them to live in comparative comfort for quite a few years. He believed that Germany would not be a good place to live for a long time, possibly even one or two decades. Before they parted company never to see each other again, and after Fritz as everyone called him, had consumed a few glasses of schnapps, he made a few observations regarding what was likely to happen in Europe in the coming years.

Even Ingrid grudgingly conceded that much if not all of what he said was most prophetic and had come to pass and also has a relevant bearing on this story.

In his view, Churchill and his cronies or backers, were insidious instigators of infamy. The view is still held by many older Germans to this very day. Although Operation Bernhard had been detected by the secret service, the economic damage to the British economy had already been accomplished. Moreover, it would probably be years before the British people were informed and would no doubt be fobbed off with a played down version of how successful this operation really was.

The true victors of the first and second world wars were not the countless millions who were killed or suffered unimaginable hardship. The real winners were the ones who actually profited. Wars are very costly and have to be financed on either side and the only ones in a position to do this are banks, multibillionaires or other financial institutions. He held, or rationalised his view and actions by believing that to steal from a thief is no crime. All he had done was to steal from a bunch of so called respectable thieves who were robbing hard working people every day. This is why he embraced the task allotted to him with such gusto. Paper money would never replace coinage made from gold, silver and other pre-cious metals. As printing techniques and photography advanced, counterfeiting paper currency would become far easier than the problems operatives of operation Bernhard had to overcome. Even-tually he said it would only be a matter of time before someone discovered or stumbled upon an alternative way of manufacturing or counterfeiting gold. After all, aluminium used to be very expen-sive until someone discovered a way that made it cheaper to manu-facture. Should such a hypothetical situation arise and he were in charge of its distribution he would call it "Operation Midas".

It was at this point Max stopped her and asked about Ulrich's father who had never been mentioned. This was quite simple, she explained. He was nothing like Ulrich's grandfather. Like many children, in spite of the love and care given to him, he grew up into a total stranger and left home as soon as he was able. This could have been due to Ilsa's radical right wing political views of which she made no secret. There must have been times when he was disturbed or even alarmed; it was very dangerous then, as now, to voice any neo-Nazi sympathies. One could be sent to prison for giving the Nazi salute.

Be that as it may, Karl got married and his wife later gave birth to a son, Ulrich. However neither Karl nor his wife was not in the least paternal or maternal to children, so Ulrich was brought up by his grandmother, who never married. Ingrid then resumed her diatribe against Ilsa. This woman, she continued, had some strange bedfellows metaphorically speaking. Right into her late eighties she maintained contact with some very unsavoury characters, mostly by letter but occasionally by telephone and the odd clandestine meeting. She had, for example, contact with the remnants of an outfit called the Baader Meinhoff gang. The activities of this notorious gang in the 1970's in Germany carried out atrocities in other countries which included bank robberies, high jacks and murders.

One of her contacts who came over from England occasionally was an elderly gentleman. He used to frequent and could have been a member of Boodles, the London club that was a backdrop for many of Ian Fleming's James Bond novels.

He (Fleming) once jokingly said that Britain had the best secret service in the world – Russia. Although it is impossible to prove, he claimed that British intelligence deliberately allowed Kim Philby, the notorious double agent responsible for the deaths of many British agents, to escape to Russia to avoid the embarrassment of putting him on trial. If this were not enough, the grandmother also received regular letters and the occasional phone call from former senior Nazi officers, or their supporters, residing in German colonies in South America. Many of these fanatics, Ingrid went on, actually believed that a fourth Reich could be created especially with the help of people like the grandmother, in other words a sort of fifth column.

Once more Max stopped her and asked her how she and Ulrich got together and what all this had to do with their relationship. Her tone suddenly changed, as though she was once again, like many of us often do, re-living some pleasant memorable event.

Ulrich was working for a large metal refining company. He was well suited to this because at university he had qualified in biochemistry and metallurgy. Consequently he was well versed in the use of spectrometers and other weird and wonderful instruments connected with metals. She herself was working as an assistant in a large jewellers shop. They met at the annual Oktoberfest, a beer festival held in Munich. She was in tears, as someone had just snatched her handbag and vanished into the crowd. Suddenly, as if by magic, Ulrich appeared and not only tried to console her, but subsequently bought her train ticket. They travelled back to Berlin together where, as luck, fate or kismet may have designated, they both resided. They fell madly in love very quickly. In a very short time they set up a home together in an apartment.

Ulrich left the home he had shared so long with his grandmother, initially with her blessing, and they lived together very happily. Then one day something happened that neither of them could have anticipated in a thousand years and finally resulted in their separation.

It was a beautiful summer's day when Ilsa received a small parcel from some Latin South American country. The contents turned out to be a very old book in Spanish printed during the eighteenth century. It was allegedly found in an old monastery and given by some kind of wise man of the mountains to one of Ilsa's Nazi friends in exile. The title comprised three words: ALQUIMIA e ORO". Translated into English it means: ALCHEMY AND GOLD. It was accompanied by a typewritten German translation. Ilsa handed the book over to Ulrich only after swearing him to secrecy, even from Ingrid. Consequently Ingrid only became aware of the matter after Ilsa had died.

A few seconds later the tape ran out so Max had to rely on his memory for the rest of Frau Schreiber's revelations. Fortunately his memory was quite retentive.

One thing was certain - this woman either had a vivid imagination or could be telling the truth. He pondered on this perplexing question for the flight. However, during his mental meanderings the same name kept recurring in his head like the opening theme of Tchaikovsky's fourth symphony. That name was Friedrick Schwend. If the man was so important in the execution of Operation Bernhard there must be some record about him and his activities somewhere. Max was determined to find out, even if it was only to satisfy his own curiosity.

At this stage it will be necessary and expedient to cover a lot of ground fast. The reason for this is because to go into all the details of certain paragraphs and even some sentences would fill a book in themselves. Consequently this work would run into several volumes. In its turn this would make the task of even attempting to read it far too daunting for the average person. The reader can draw their own conclusions as to whether this work is the ramblings of some crank who doesn't know what he is talking about. So, we will now move on, but at a slightly faster pace.

## Chapter 13
## Meltdown

We will come to the exact circumstances that led to the separation of Ingrid and Ulrich in due course. In the meantime a few words about alchemy are in order.

Over the centuries, men have tried to find the process in which base metals could be transformed into gold – alchemy. None of these have succeeded as far as we know, and even if they had it would most certainly not be in the interests of the one's who achieved this accomplishment to advertise their achievements. During the Middle Ages it was an occupational hazard to have one's house burned down even if it was only rumoured one was practising alchemy.

However, one little known case that occurred in Southall, London in 1935 is worthy of a mention. Charles Gladitz was born in Germany in 1866 but arrived in England in 1922, from        Mozambique. He had travelled first class with his wife, and the couple moved into 6 Gunnersberg Avenue and settled into    local life. Gladitz was a research chemist and ended up on the board of directors at a company called The New Process Company Limited. Founded in 1931, the company had a factory in Scotts Road, Southall. It was here that Gladitz began his mysterious work. He claimed to be working on a process where volcanic lava could be transformed into gold. He said he could make £50,000,000 per year, and the money given to the treasury to reduce the national debt and levels of income tax. Reginald McKenna, the chairman of Midland Bank, seemed to take the matter seriously, judging from some correspondence between the two men. Unfortunately they did not get the opportunity of meeting in person to discuss the matter further, and resolving the national problem. Gladitz suddenly committed suicide.

The circumstances of his untimely death were as mysterious or questionable as those surrounding the apparent suicide of Dr David Kelly, the weapons expert. This it will be recalled was just before Tony Blair dragged us into the war against Iraq; also Gladitz's notes and papers suddenly disappeared and were never found.

We will now return to what led to the separation of Ingrid Schreiber and Ulrich. It was a few months when, after finishing work, Ulrich decided to call on his grandmother on his way back home. He told her that he had been working in his laboratory. He then produced something interesting to show her what he had been working on for several weeks, handing his grandmother a bar which he had removed from his pocket, it was a small bar, which looked like it could be gold. Her initial reaction was that it felt very heavy for its size and asked him if it was real gold. Shaking his head and smiling to himself he told her it was not, it was just a good imitation. He then quickly added that just to put his handy work to the test, so to speak, he had taken it to several jewellers and said she would never believe what happened next. At this point he said his throat was getting dry and asked if she would get him a cold beer. By now Ilsa burning with curiosity and with trembling hands poured him his beer and asked him to continue.

Speaking with an air of modest pride, he told her that not only did they weigh it, file it and gave it the acid test, but they offered to buy it for several hundred Euros. It was quite obvious they believed it to be gold. (Incidentally, a similar thing happened when Max carried out his own test a few weeks later. Two of the coins given to him in   India were passed off as genuine by some of the best numismatists in Europe)

Ulrich tried to illicit some information about the old Spanish book she had given him for his perusal some time ago. Ilsa simply brushed the question aside, poured herself a rather large schnapps that would make many people insensible and looked very serious. After swearing him to secrecy yet again, and not to breathe a word about their meeting to Ingrid, she asked him if she could borrow his recent acquisition, adding that she would take good care of it. She then asked him if he would drop in and see her, on his own, about the same time the following week. The reason for this being there was someone she would like him to meet. With that they parted company.

When he arrived the next week he was introduced to an elderly, very distinguished looking gentleman in his seventies or early eighties. We will call this gentleman Werner. Now, Ulrich was uncertain what this meeting was going to be about but Werner came straight to the point by asking a few direct questions.

Would he, Ulrich, like to deliver a devastating blow to the biggest enemies of not only the German people but also most of Europe? Before he had time to gather his thoughts and answer, Werner quickly followed up by asking him if it would be possible to manufacture his imitation gold on a much bigger scale, but in coinage rather than small bars? It was the second question that prompted a quick answer from Ulrich. Shaking his head he said it would be possible but highly improbable as far as he was concerned.

He continued that an undertaking of this magnitude would require a much larger laboratory than that in which he worked. Apart from good quality sample coins to be used as prototypes, possibly specialist engravers and even a special workshop and a small scale factory would be necessary. All of these facilities were not, or even likely to be at his disposal in Germany.

Werner listened very attentively to everything that had been said to him. He then sat back in his chair and asked Ilsa, who had also been sitting quietly, to get them a drink. What followed must have sounded like part of the screenplay of that famous film: The Godfather. Just suppose he could wave a zauberstab, (magicians wand) and all these facilities, along with a house and at least two servants, plus a salary of three times the amount he was currently earning, Would this idea appeal to him even if only in the name of science?

It would entail him re-locating to another country in the Middle East and he could take Ingrid with him, but he must only tell her that he had the offer of a better job working with metals, which was about as true as he could make it.

One thing led to another and an agreement was reached but Ingrid preferred to remain in Germany. Nevertheless she agreed to let him give it a try, fully confident he would be dying to come back to his beloved Germany within three months.

Well he wasn't and didn't, and although they kept in touch and met up from time to time in India or some other warm climate, it was the death knell of their relationship. This is why Ingrid felt such en-mity against Ulrich's grandmother.

Chapter 14
The Search


The first item on Max's agenda upon returning to the UK was to glean any information he could about Friedrich Schwend and the alleged major part he played in "Operation Bernhard". To this end he galvanised his internet scouts and other contacts to find out all they could. Whilst he was waiting for the results of their enquiries he made a few investigations in other directions himself. He subsequently uncovered some snippets of information of which the British Public were unaware and were never told, even at the time of this publication.

A senior spokesman for one of the biggest British coin and banknote dealers informed him that the five pound notes were not the biggest headache which faced the Bank of England. What really concerned them was the possibility, even probability, that they may well be prints of ten shilling and pound notes that would attract little if any attention, especially if they were of the same high standard of the high denomination notes. In anticipation of such a contingency arising, the board game and playing card manufacturers John Waddington's, based in Wakefield Yorkshire were put on standby to print replacement notes. Fortunately, as events turned out this was not necessary. In the meantime Max's internet scouts had checked everything that was available on all relevant websites. One of his team managed to get all the episodes of a T.V. series called Private Schultz that was broadcast in the 1970's or 80's starring Michael Elphick. It was a comedy that was loosely based on Operation Bernhard. There were also other fictional films available and Max not only watched every-one, he read every printout that had come off the internet.

Although the names of many senior Nazi officers were incorporated into the stories, the name he was so desperately searching for was as elusive as Lord Lucan. He began to wonder if the whole story was simply a figment of Frau Schreider's imagination. The only flaw with this theory however, was the small matter of the coins that were in his possession. No person in their right mind would give about ten thousand pounds, in genuine gold coins, to have their fortune told, and whatever his former German acquaintance was, she was by no means a lunatic.

Most investigators, at some time or other, reach a stage in their progression when they feel that cannot go any further and are about to give up when they get a break. Max was no exception. One evening he received a telephone call from one of his team who seemed to spend most of her time browsing in charity shops. She excitedly told him she had stumbled across a fairly old book published in the United States in 1961 entitled Operation Bernhard by someone called Anthony Pirie. It contained several photographs including one of Friedrich Schwend.

The Power of Books

> Throughout history, priests, politicians, bigots, dictators and any organisation or state that has depended on total conformity, have always recognised and dreaded the power of books. They have banned, suppressed, confiscated and burned them, their authors, printers, distributors and readers have been threatened with ridicule, exposure, disgrace, torture, excommunication or even death. For books can kindle dreams, wither bigotry, shatter illusions, change people's ideas and topple empires.
> ©Peter Gill

As soon as it arrived in the post and the parcel opened, Max held it with feverish hands and read it from cover to cover. It is probably the most comprehensive account of this aspect of the Second World War ever published.

Frau Schreiber was certainly not exaggerating in her account of Friedrich Schwend's role in Operation Bernhard. Quite the        contrary, if anything she was being quite conservative. It was most unlikely that she could have read the book in question as it was published, and been out of print before she was even born.

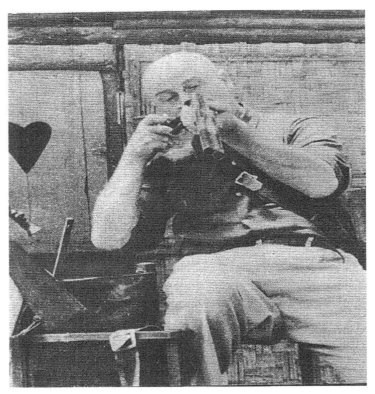

Friedrich Schwend In Peru in the 1960s

# Chapter 15

## Operation Bernhard – The Untold Story

Contrary to what we have been led to believe, it was in fact the British who unwittingly created Operation Bernhard and indirectly, over half a century later, Operation Midas.

Very briefly this is how it happened.

At the beginning of the Second World War the RAF dropped tens of thousands of counterfeit clothing coupons over various German cities. This turned out to be a foolhardy move that was made as a result of false or bad intelligence, because clothing was not yet rationed. Later they tried dropping counterfeit two Reichmark notes but they were so bad that the German people simply handed them in to the police. This must have triggered off the concept of a similar but more elaborate operation, albeit carried out with Teutonic efficiency against the British. Although this is what subsequently happened, there were many setbacks and false starts before it finally got underway, but every single one was overcome.

When the idea was first propounded at a high level Nazi conference it was received with a mixture of laughter, horror and scepticism, mostly the latter, especially by Walter Funk, the minister of finance. For simplicity an outline of the principle reasons as to why such a hair-brained scheme could never work, is as follows:

Even if it were possible to produce such banknotes, to drop them all over England would be totally impracticable. They would very quickly attract so much attention that the whole operation would be halted almost before it began. How would these miraculous banknotes going to be distributed? There was also the problem of the paper. This was made from special rag that could only be obtained from India, of which the British had total dominion since the eighteenth century.

In addition to the foregoing there was the problem of the numbering system, of which only the Bank of England was privy. Every banknote from five pounds upwards was registered, and if any note did not correspond to the date, years of circulation and number on the note in question, payment would be refused and the whole plan would collapse like a house of cards. Incidentally, once again it must be remembered that five, ten, twenty and fifty pounds was worth far more than it is at the time of this publication.

Even nowadays many traders in the UK will not accept fifty pound notes. In some poorer countries of Europe like Spain, if one tenders a one hundred Euro note (about £80) many traders and bars, especially smaller ones, will insist on only accepting smaller denominations. To return to Operation Bernhard, It is now time to introduce the three protagonists responsible for its success.

Initially Reinhard Heydrich, head of the all powerful security services, and one of the most feared men in Germany, was put in charge of Operation Bernhard. Along with a man called Bernhard Kruger, who we will come to presently, they scoured all the concentration camps and prisons in Germany and Poland for every forger, engraver and other miscellanies criminals who had ever made a dishonest living. They were all rounded up and put in Blocks 18 & 19 in Sachsenhausen concentration camp, north of Berlin, each were given extra special rations and other privileges to carry out the tasks allotted to them. Unfortunately, (depending on which side one is on) Heydrich was assassinated by Czech patriots in Prague on the 28th May 1942. He was replaced by Walter Schellenberg, who proved to be far more imaginative. By the way, Schellenberg was one of the few defendants who were acquitted at the Nuremberg trials in 1946.

We now come to Bernhard Kruger. This man, a former textile engineer, was the chief forger of passports and other important documents, his knowledge and expertise were invaluable. Last but not least we come to Friedrich Schwend, who solved the problem of distribution in a way, with the benefit of hindsight, was so simple but also turned out to be highly effective. To this end we must profile this man and his career, even before he became involved in Operation Bernhard.

Friedrich Schwend was a big time German business man who settled at the Italian luxury seaside resort of Abbazia after an adventurous exciting life. While still a garage mechanic in Swabia, he had married a local aristocratic heiress and then acted as a representative for various firms. Later he was invited to California by his wife's aunt, who like her, had married against the family wishes. The widowed and extremely wealthy aunt was so impressed by Schwend's personal charm and business ability that she gave him sole power of attorney to manage her fortune in the United States, Argentina, Switzerland and elsewhere. Schwend now extended his business experience all over the world. He worked in South America, and helped to organise an efficient provisioning system in Russia during Lenin's new economic policy period, and made various trips to China. He also met the white Russian Commander, General Seminoff, for whom he obtained arms by the shiploads. Early in the 1930's he returned to Germany and rapidly recognised the latent dangers in the Nazi "self – sufficiency" economic policy. He offered his services as consultant, and his advice impressed Goering. The Gestapo, however, suspected that a much travelled cosmopolite like Schwend might be an enemy agent. Gestapo agents searched Schwend's house so he went to America, and as a precaution, on his return to Europe at the outbreak of war, settled in Abbazia, where he had a luxurious villa and a yacht.

Now, one of the agents who were active in the distribution of these fake British notes was a man called Fröben. Fröben was introduced by Schwend to many of his contacts. These included important industrialists, ship owners and other wealthy people interested in buying foreign currency. This not only enabled Fröben to make big sales, but also to pick up valuable information. One day, in a casual talk to Schwend he said "if we had a political intelligence service, it would pay any price for what I have learned selling these pounds" these words sparked off a big business idea in Schwend's mind.

Schwend suggested that the forged pounds should be turned out by the millions and used to finance German intelligence work throughout the world. Also, a little known fact was that Germany had very little foreign currency and the Reichmark was only valid in German occupied territory. But pounds sterling were and still are accepted all over the world. Fröben thought it a brilliant idea and said he ought to put it to Schellenberg, which he did, and it was eventually acted upon.

From this moment Operation Bernhard began to take off in a really big way. All foreign Nazi agents were paid generously with forged notes. As they had already passed the ultimate test by being accepted as genuine by the Bank of England, they could be tendered with impunity and exchanged for any foreign currency outside German occupied territory.

The British were in fact unwittingly paying for valuable information and intelligence that was being given to their enemies. Perhaps one of their most audacious stunts, apart from spending tens of thousands of "pounds" in bribes to facilitate the rescue of Mussolini by Otto Scorceny, it was the purchase of arms, supplied by the British to allied partisans and then used to fight the very people who had supplied them.

The foregoing is only a summary of an event in history that would otherwise occupy several hundred pages and there were obviously many other people involved. However, It probably goes without saying that Schwend became a key player in Operation Bernhard exactly as Frau Schreiber had claimed on that warm December evening in India back in 2011. Whether there is any truth in the theory of hereditary is debateable, but if Ulrich was anything like his grandfather, he must have been, and possibly still is, quite an extraordinary man. All this of course was hushed up and played down, even after the Second World War had long ended.

Just before closing on Operation Bernhard, a few words about what finally happened to the three protagonists who were responsible for its success are in order.

Walter Schellenberg died in 1952 aged 48.

Bernard Kruger worked for the post-war German Government as a consultant on rural housing finance. Friedrich Schwend fled to South America and lived a quiet life in Lima Peru. However, he had managed to acquire a considerable fortune. The following is only what is on record and documented:

He had 1,500,000 Francs in the Vaduz branch of the Bank of Lichtenstein, a holding worth another million Swiss Francs in a Trieste property company, a holding worth 350,000 Marks in an Austrian import and export firm, and nearly 100,000 Marks worth of securities – all earned as a sales director for Operation Bernhard.

We will now move on to Operation Midas.

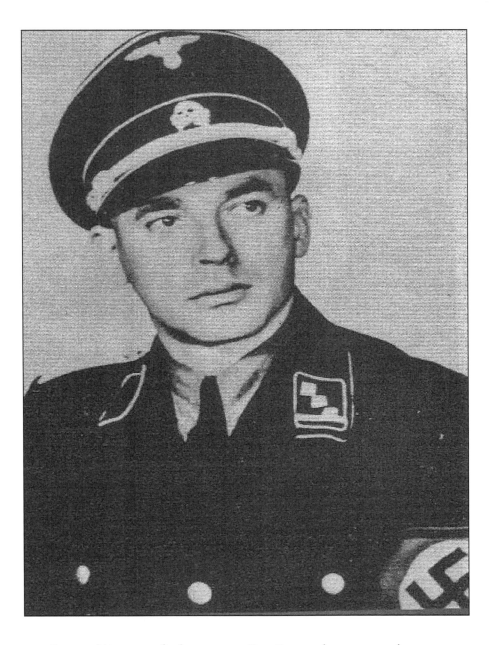

Bernard Kruger, of whom operation Bernard was named, was a former textile engineer, and was the chief forger of Passports and other documents

# Chapter 16
## Operation Midas

The old adage that nobody is indispensable may well be true but there are some people who are very difficult, if not almost impossible to replace.

Every time we look at our television we seldom if ever give a thought to the man who made it possible. During the time John Logie Baird worked on his invention, the insurance premiums on his life were astronomical. The reason for this was simple. There was nobody else on this planet that had his knowledge or expertise who could replace him. His financial backers recognised this and did not want to take any chances with their investment. Being shrewd businessmen they no doubt perceived or realised that they were onto something that would revolutionise entertainment, and they were right, even though it did not happen overnight.

A similar situation probably occurred with Ulrich, albeit for totally different reasons and motives. Exactly how much of Ulrich's gold was and may still be being made is impossible to assess. On a T.V. broadcast, a small factory in the West Midlands that was churning out counterfeit one pound coins by the thousands every week was exposed. Distribution of coins of such a small denomination hardly raised an eyebrow. Even banks barely gave them a second glance, which is probably why one in three in current circulation is counterfeit. But gold coins in theory, is a different matter, or is it?

The logistics and feasibility of distributing large quantities of gold in Europe is not as daunting or farfetched as it may first appear. For one thing Europe is not at war and border controls in EEU countries are virtually none existent.

One of Max's contacts travelled by car from England to France and then drove down to Italy to where he was re-locating. He was carrying over one hundred thousand pounds in gold sovereigns. (Genuine ones it must be added) he not only went unmolested, but was not asked for his passport on either side of the English Channel. In addition to this, in the UK the authorities are already fighting a losing battle against illegal immigrants and the import of counterfeit cigarettes, not to mention drugs, so what chance do they have against the odd kilo of gold coins?

Travel by air, at least in Europe, is equally safe, if one can tolerate the long queues and being searched for weapons. It is true that if one is found in possession of ten thousand or more Euros', and does not declare it, they have a good chance of having it confiscated. However, carrying coins poses no such problems. On many occasions Max himself has been in possession of twenty or thirty thousand pounds worth of valuable coins that are kept in a small album that fits in his pocket. He was once stopped at Manchester airport on his way to Gibraltar but the official simply looked at them, admired them and gave them back.

Selling gold in all shapes and forms has never posed a problem to the ones who have it. Although traders are supposed to be shown some proof of identity, especially during large transactions of over five thousand pounds and most do carry out this practice. However, it must be remembered that dodgy, greedy and unscrupulous traders are not just confined to the used car industry. Also most jewellers will gladly accept gold coins in part exchange for some piece of antique jewellery or diamond ring etc. that is authentic. This same principle also applies to many pawnbrokers who are also jewellers.

Auction houses are also very good outlets for the disposal of coins of all sizes, ages, denominations and countries, even though the commission charged to both the seller and the buyer is considered by many as exorbitant.

In view of the foregoing, if Operation Midas was being executed on similar lines to Operation Bernhard, as Max had good reason to believe it was and still is, it does not take much of a leap of reason and imagination to perceive the ramifications of this scenario. In addition to this, even if only as few as twenty well trained agents who were well versed in what has just been outlined and probably much more besides were active, it should be of much concern to the treasury, at least worthy of an enquiry. It has long been the policy of intelligence agencies to regard information that has been easily obtained to be of little or no value. Rather like the old adage: "offered services stink". This kind of attitude has, throughout history, caused the needless cost of many lives.

Just to give a couple of examples, taken from many, from both sides of the Second World War should illustrate what Max means.

Shortly before Norway entered the Second World War, a document which later became known as The Oslo Report, was delivered anonymously to the British Embassy in Norway. It was purported to have been compiled by a scientist. Among many other things it contained details of weapons which the Germans had already developed, or were in the process of developing. These included the V1 and V2 rockets which were the first ground to air missiles, and the Messerschmitt 262, the world's first jet fighter.

This document was sent to London to be examined by the boffins who did not take it seriously, at least initially. It was only when the allies began to suffer the effects of some of the weapons that they had already been warned about, when they began to sit up and take notice.

The second example is taken from the axis or German side, and was immortalized in a film made in about 1952 starring James Mason entitled "5 Fingers" This incident took place during 1944 in Ankara, Turkey, a neutral country. It was called Operation Cicero. The valet to the British Ambassador was an Albanian who had been in service for some years with certain members of the aristocracy. He approached the attaché at the German Embassy and offered to sell his government photographs of British top secret documents. For the sum of one hundred and fifty thousand pounds, he subsequently sold the Nazi's hundreds of top secret documents which included the allied plans for operation overlord. He gave the date and all the details of the Normandy landings scheduled for the 5th or 6th of June 1944. This was vital intelligence indeed, by then the war was going very badly for Germany and Field Marshall Rommel warned Hitler that if he couldn't push the invasion back into the sea he would lose the war. Unfortunately, although Franz- Von Papen believed the documents were genuine, a man called Kaltenbrunner, the head of the gestapo thought they were just a trap planted by the British. As he out ranked Franz-Von Papen, the German Ambassador, in authority he refused to act on the plethora of priceless information that had been handed to him for virtually nothing. Nothing being the operative word, because they paid their informant with forged banknotes from Operation Bernhard.

However he did not discover this until he had fled to Rio-de Janerio.

The last two incidents just related had a special irony in the final chapter of this story however. Just before arriving at the climax of what began as an exotic holiday, a few words about the law and counterfeit coins are in order.

To manufacture sovereigns, guineas or any other coins that are no longer in circulation, out of imitation gold is no crime in itself. It is also not illegal to sell them providing the seller states exactly what they are. If however you try to pass them off as genuine you could find yourself in big trouble. It is sad but true to say that some dealers and even auction houses must sometimes have serious doubts about certain items that pass through their hands. When this occurs, to cover themselves, they are simply described "As seen". Some people actually collect counterfeit coins, jewellery and other items. Not for fraudulent purposes it must be hastily added, but to illustrate what serious collectors can be up against.

In short it is simply a case of "let the buyer beware". We will now move on to the conclusion of a story that started in India and ended in Vienna.

## Chapter 17
## Strauss, Schnitzel & Satisfaction

To go into detail of what some people would call the seedy James Bond world of the crooked gold industry, as stated earlier, would occupy more space than it deserves. However, to give the reader an idea of at least part of what Max's subsequent, not to mention expensive investigation revealed is worthy of inclusion in this work.

Max interviewed many honest and dodgy coin and bullion dealers. Some of which were secretly recorded on a micro cassette recorder. These comprised people from four countries in Europe in addition to the UK and Gibraltar. Several of the latter admitted buying up to twenty of the same large denomination coins allegedly minted in Mexico, Spain, Cuba, France, the United States and the UK. All of which were purchased well below the standard price of gold at that particular time and with no questions asked about the source of origin.

One dodgy dealer, after a few drinks and a large meal paid for by Max, openly boasted of being supplied regularly since 2009. When questioned about the person who supplied him, he replied that it was a man of Middle Eastern appearance in his mid to late thirties. Then, looking furtively from side to side, almost whispered that the coins were copies but made from real gold that the Germans had managed to get out of the country just before the end of the Second World War. Max secretly thought to himself that even though this explanation was highly unlikely, it was the best cover story he had heard. Be that as it may, over a period of two years max amassed a huge dossier of irrefutable evidence that would convince the most ardent sceptic that Operation Midas was no fairy tale.

Quite naturally he felt this was of national importance, especially to the treasury and gold industry. He also felt that even a corrupt politician would at least call for an enquiry. How wrong he turned out to be.

He wrote to two leading politicians who he believed to be men of integrity but didn't even get a reply. It might be added that he wrote to them at their home address and not to the House of Commons. He later quipped that it should be re-named the house of traitors. His next step was writing to the editors of some of the leading newspapers. Once again he never received a reply. As a last resort, Max telephoned several newspapers and spoke to some excuses for journalists. He explained that he had a good story that he was not prepared to discuss over the phone, but if they came to see him they would not be disappointed. They promised to call him back but didn't.

However, there was one journalist who did take the trouble to come and see him which raised his hopes. During their meeting max told the journalist about himself, his many contacts and gave him a brief outline of Operation Midas in the presence of a witness of the highest integrity. Unfortunately, the reporter only seemed interested in a notorious criminal who had recently died, he was one of Max's former clients and the reporter ran a feature on this issue. There was another man who had, intently or not, swindled many people out of millions of pounds and who was still at large. This issue resulted in another feature, but once again the journalist was not interested in pursuing Operation Midas.

Some men would have given up in despair but Max firmly believed that you only fail when you stop trying.

Ideas and inspirations can come into one's head at the most unexpected and sometimes awkward moments. It was such a circumstance that prompted Max to take what was not only his last chance of getting any further in finding someone to examine the findings of his investigation, but also what seemed his last hope too.

One evening he was clearing out some old papers and letters. He stumbled across a photograph of one of his many contacts he had made friends with on one of his European trips. We will call him Otto. Now Otto was a retired former KGB agent who worked in what used to be East Germany with Vladimir Putin until 1989 and the collapse of communism. As a front he worked as a correspondent for a prestigious West German magazine and lived in Vienna, which was where Max met him. They had shared some very pleasant evenings together along with good beer.

By the way, one does not have to be Russian to belong to the KGB any more than one has to be British to belong to MI6. Most intelligence agencies employ foreign nationals if they can prove their worth by supplying important and credible information.

One of the many men Max interviewed was a man called John Symonds; this person is no fictitious character. Scotland Yard will have a file on him but it's most unlikely they would make it public. John was a former Scotland Yard officer who became so appalled at the corruption in his department that he tried to do something about it. Fortunately for him he got wind that he was about to be fit up and sent to prison so he fled, initially to Europe. He subsequently came to the attention of the KGB and agreed to be one of their numbers. He felt that they couldn't be any worse than the outfit he had just left so he became a fully-fledged agent.

Alas, like many ex-pats who seek refuge abroad, (like David Shaylor, a former whistle-blower from MI6 who Max also interviewed) he probably became homesick and returned to Britain and was sent to prison for two years. When Max interviewed John he was in the process of writing a book entitled "Dirty Secrets" but died before it was completed.

Getting back to Otto, Perhaps Max was tackling this story from the wrong angle, after all the idea was German originally, perhaps they might be interested. To this end he contacted Otto and, after exchanging pleasantries outlined Operation Midas and asked him, through the "old Boy" network, if he would put out a few feelers to see if his former editor would be interested.

A few days later Max received a call from Otto asking him if he actually had any of the coins in question, and if he had would he send a couple so they could be tested, possibly to destruction. Max promptly despatched one coin from Operation Midas and a genuine sovereign, but at that stage did not disclose this. About another week went by and Max received a call from Otto. He said that the experts had found an irregularity with one of the coins, When Max asked which one it was, and given the date, it turned out to be the genuine sovereign with which they had found the irregularity. It was pretty obvious that they couldn't tell which was which and it could have been a bluff.

When Max explained this to Otto he sounded non-plussed and said he would get back to him. Within two hours Max received another call from Otto and this time he sounded quite excited. His former editor was most interested and if Max had anymore coins and was willing to bring them, along with all the evidence he had amassed, a meeting could be arranged anywhere in Europe which Max cared to designate.

Now Max usually attended the annual international Numismatic fair that was held in Vienna each year in April. This incidentally was one of the many outlets for the disposal of coins from Operation Midas, and usually with no questions asked.

A meeting was arranged for the 25$^{th}$ April 2014 at a location on the Mariahilfer Strasse, not far from where the hotel where Max usually stayed during his visits. Otto cautioned him and said that he would be subject to severe questioning, especially regarding any persons he many have discussed the matter with, and journalists in particular. He may even have to submit to undergoing a lie detector test. As things worked out, this turned out to be unnecessary. His evidence was so overwhelming and he presented the facts so cogently that it was obvious he knew what he was talking about, although he did have to make an affidavit. (Part of which is reproduced later in this chapter) Just before settling the final details Max brought up the unpleasant subject of money.

This investigation had been very expensive with the cost of airline tickets, hotel bills and other incidental expenses, unlike Rupert Murdoch, who practically owned the news industry and had his lackeys all over the world; Max was one man band who only had the help of what he called citizen journalists. If this enterprise paid off he intended to pay them all for their efforts. Otto himself was to be paid one thousand  Euros' for his service so he was not talking about a few hundred Euro's.  Max named the figure that he wanted that was firm, fast and non-negotiable. If the magazine in question didn't want it then he would simply lick his wounds and put the whole thing down to experience. And he meant it. His concern and apprehension turned out to be groundless. The meeting went without a hitch, except for the task of swearing an affidavit, part of which is reproduced here:

**"Part 4 of Affidavit made by Max 25-04-2014**

*The only journalist I have ever spoken to about the aforementioned subject is a man, whose name I prefer not to reveal, and works for a provincial national newspaper. However, as he is only in possession of a fraction of the facts and information I have related, he poses no threat to making public this exposition, and I will explain why.*

*After writing to several politicians and news editors and receiving no response, I tried telephoning a few fellow journalists who, in the past, I have furnished with reliable information that was newsworthy.*

*Eventually I managed to speak to the above mentioned person and during our conversation I told him about my connection with a notorious criminal who had recently died. This journalist subsequently came to see me on the 6th January this year. As a result of our conversation, he did a feature on that story that was syndicated worldwide.*

*However, in the presence of a witness of the highest integrity, I gave him a brief summary of "Operation Midas" only after he gave me an undertaking that if he used the information he would not reveal the source of it. This was because, I explained, I did not want to spend eternity propping up some motorway. He said he would check it out when he had time, but deep down I felt that he didn't show the enthusiasm I had hoped or expected. I later gave him information about a notorious fraudster who had swindled many people out of millions of pounds and, at the time of this statement being prepared, is still at large.*

*Actually it was this man's name, among other dodgy bullion dealer's that cropped up during my two years investigation into "Operation Midas".*

*This resulted in another feature that was syndicated worldwide and, although I am not a materialist and do not need the money, even out of common courtesy I never received a single penny from that newspaper.*

*Be that as it may, I arranged to spend an evening with this journalist along with his wife. This was because, by and large, women are far more intuitive than men, and if I outlined further details, not to mention the ramifications of "Operation Midas" and the tenuous connection to "Operation Bernhard", which is well documented. His wife may well have perceived exactly what was being handed to her husband on a platter. Unfortunately she could not attend I discovered when I got to the arranged meeting place, so I had simply wasted my time, and was secretly disappointed.*

*To be perfectly fair to the man, he is a dedicated journalist and good at his job. But having said that, he probably would not thank me for saying the following, I am of the firm opinion that a man of his calibre is being exploited by his employer and would be far better setting up his own news agency, as I did in 1997, at the age fifty nine.*

*Also, to give the man more credit, he is a crime reporter, and a competent one at that. However, when it comes to criminal activities by certain governments at the highest level by their intelligence agencies of which you gentlemen are familiar, not to mention metaphysics, occultism and certain esoteric subjects, he is definitely out of his depth.*

*I think I have now answered all your questions which have been backed up by evidence in your possession. I have nothing further to add to this statement, which has been voluntary.*


*Signed Max*

*25-04 2014 Vienna"*


Although he was paid in full, it was in 500 Euro notes. This posed a slight but not insurmountable problem. Back in the UK Thomas Cook would not even change a 100 Euro note. However, at the coin fair that was taking place here in Vienna, they were changing hands like five pound notes in any public house or shop in the UK. The answer was simple. He would just buy a few high value gold coins that he knew were not being manufactured by Operation Midas. This is      exactly what he did. Incidentally, for some rea-son Russian gold coins, with the exception of 37.5 Rouble, which is quite scarce      and German, Chinese and certain gold coins from the Middle East were not being manufactured by Operation Midas.

Max enjoyed the rest of his stay in Vienna. He went to the opera, a Strauss concert in the Stadpark, and was ready to return home. This is where the story could end. But there was a final twist that Max could never have imagined.

On the evening before his departure back to the UK, he met up with Otto for a few beers and a little farewell celebration. It was on this memorable evening that Otto dropped his bombshell.

It turned out that the magazine he used to work for was not interested in his story. Operation Bernhard was an aspect of German history they did not wish to regurgitate, and Operation Midas was even worse. However, Otto knew some people who would be very interested and would willingly pay what he asked without a quibble. To this end, he arranged the meeting that went successfully a few evenings ago.

At this point Max started to get a most uneasy feeling. His intuition told him to raise his hand and stop Otto before he uttered another syllable. He suspected what was about to follow but did not want his suspicions confirmed.

For months Max had been trying to get someone to listen to him and felt rather like a pedlar selling clockwork toys. At long last he had found somebody, regardless of their creed, colour, nationality, religious, or political persuasion to recognise what was being presented to them. If it meant doing a deal with the devil himself and Otto was Mephistopheles and this was act three of Faust, then so be it. He did what he thought was right. Just before they parted company, Otto made a casual remark that rang in Max's ears:

"Whys is it that the British always learn when it is too late".

We are now at the end of the story but a few words of wisdom or even caution are offered to any reflective person:

Ideas cannot be killed any more than trying to put a genie back in a bottle. Knowledge and real history can only be suppressed for a limited time.

In short:

> *For nothing is secret, that shall not be made manifest; neither anything hid, that shall not be known and come abroad.*

> St Luke 8 verse 17

> PEACE TO ALL WHO READ THESE LINES.

Mit ihrer Art und Vielfalt des Angebots die größte Münzen-Messe der Welt mit unverkennbarem Flair und gepflegter Tradition seit 1970!

## Messeangebote:

Münzen und Medaillen von der Antike bis Heute, Papiergeld, Wertpapiere, Fachliteratur und Zubehör

With its style and variety of offerings, the world's biggest coin fair with distinctive flair and refined tradition since 1970!

## Fair Exhibits:

ancient and modern coins, medals, paper money, bond certificates, literature, accessories

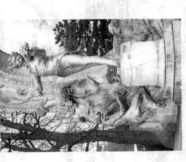

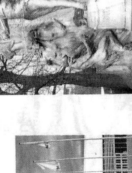

**2014**

The International Numismatic Fair

NUMISMATA ®

Wien. Austria

seit 1970